DIABETES: A NEW GUIDE

Rowan Hillson
MD MRCP

Illustrated by
Maggie Raynor

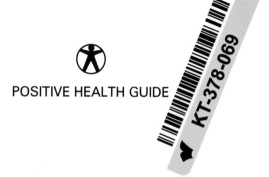

POSITIVE HEALTH GUIDE

Dedication
For those who live with diabetes

An OPTIMA Book

Copyright © Rowan Hillson 1992

The right of Dr Rowan Hillson to be identified as
author of this work has been asserted by
her in accordance with the Copyright, Designs
and Patents Act 1988.

First published in 1992 by Optima
Reprinted 1993, 1994

A CIP catalogue record for this
book is available from the
British Library

Typeset in 10pt Parlament by Leaper & Gard Ltd, Bristol
Printed and bound in Great Britain by
the Alden Press, Oxford

Optima Books
A Division of
Little, Brown and Company (UK)
Brettenham House
Lancaster Place
London WC2E 7EN

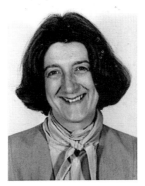

Rowan Hillson, MD, MRCP is a Consultant Physician with a special interest in Diabetes at The Hillingdon Hospital, Middlesex. She wrote her first book about diabetes while working in Oxford where she completed several diabetes research projects. Now she shares the care of several thousand people with diabetes with other members of the Hillingdon Diabetes Team. Dr Hillson is an enthusiast of outdoor activities and several times a year she takes groups of diabetics of all ages on Outward Bound courses. She works closely with the British Diabetic Association, and has a particular interest in helping people with diabetes to learn more about their condition. She is the author of *Diabetes Beyond 40, Diabetes: A Young Person's Guide* and *Diabetes: A Beyond Basics Guide, Diabetes: A New Guide,* and *Thyroid Disorders,* all published by Optima.

Also by Dr Rowan Hillson in the Positive Health Guides series:
Beyond Basics Guide
Diabetes Beyond 40
Diabetes: A Young Person's Guide
Diabetes: A New Guide
Thyroid Disorders

CONTENTS

ACKNOWLEDGEMENTS

This book would not have been written without the constant stimulus and enthusiasm of the people with diabetes I have known over the years. I thank them for sharing their diabetes with me.

I am very grateful to the following for their help, ideas, comments, encouragement and support:

Jayne Booth, The British Diabetic Association, Brenda Cox, The Hillingdon Diabetes Team, Kay and Rodney Hillson, Simon Hillson, Margaret Hounslow, Richard Hourston, Hugh Mather, Richenda Milton-Thompson, David Perkin, Suzanne Redmond, Kate Smallman, Yvonne Stawarz, Peter Thompson, Clare Wallis.

Maggie Raynor converted my drawings into illustrations. Photograph by Yvonne Hollis.

I would also like to thank the following for their permission to use material reproduced in this book:

Colin Duncan and MIMS for the table of insulins on page 84 taken from the December 1991 edition (n.b. this chart is up-dated in each month's issue of MIMS); the Journal of the Royal College of Physicians of London for the table shown on page 70 taken from Volume 17, no. 1 of January, 1983; The British Diabetic Association for 'What diabetic care to expect' on page 208 and 'What professional supervision should children with diabetes and their families expect?'; International Diabetes Federation (Europe) and the Editor and publishers (John Wiley and Sons Ltd) of Diabetic Medicine for The St Vincent Declaration (Diabetic Medicine 1990: 7: 360) and the European Patients' Charter (Diabetic Medicine 1991: 8: 782-3); University of Toronto Press for extracts from Living with Diabetes by Heather Maclean and Barbara Oram, 1988 (page 162).

To maintain your health it is not enough that your doctor should put you on the proper lines of treatment. You must learn to follow it and carry it out yourself in your own home. This alone will insure your health and give you a mastery over the disease and liberty to carry on your usual life.

R.D. Lawrence, 1935
(Co-founder of the British Diabetic Association)

FOREWORD

A diagnosis of diabetes hits people with an awful force. Suddenly no longer a person but a 'patient', life is suddenly filled with questions. Will I need injections every day? Must I stop eating my favourite foods? Can I have children? Am I now a sick person? Dare I go on holiday? And, always, who or what's to blame? Is there a cure? Is life going to be worth living?

While these questions crowd in most of all on the newly diagnosed person, they also besiege parents, partners, relatives and friends. They are questions that must be answered for life to be as full and complete, as gratifying and productive as it was before. This new book aims to answer these questions.

This is a helpful and hopeful book. It tackles all the key questions fully and frankly and in a way that all of those with, or living with, diabetes can understand. It will be a valuable aid to the essential process of understanding and coming to terms with diabetes, a process in which doctors, nurses, members of the 'diabetes care team' and other people with diabetes all play an important part.

The book opens with a quotation from perhaps the most remarkable diabetic patient of them all, the redoubtable Dr R D Lawrence. He not only wrote a classic book *The Diabetic Life* – he also lived it to the full. His major memorial is the British Diabetic Association which he founded and which offers its support and a welcome to all members of this club that nobody wanted to join.

Harry Keen
Emeritus Professor of Human Metabolism
Guy's Hospital, London
Chairman, Executive Council, British Diabetic Association
Hon. President, International Diabetes Federation

INTRODUCTION

This book is for people who have just learned that they have diabetes, for their relatives and carers, and for people who have had diabetes for some time but would like some revision.

One in one hundred people has diabetes and knows it. We all know someone who has diabetes – someone in the family, a friend, someone at work. One person in a hundred has diabetes and does not realise that they have it. People will have diabetes without you being aware of it – for people with diabetes look no different from anyone else, and can work and have fun just like anyone else.

But having it yourself is different. Until it has been treated it can make you feel off colour or very ill. And it is always frightening when you discover that something is wrong with you. It is especially frightening if you do not know anything about this new condition. As a small child I was always told to be very, very careful with electricity. If I wasn't, I would get a shock. Everyone kept telling me how careful I must be. So I thought that a shock must be very, very dangerous. Then one day, as I plugged in the iron, I had a small electric shock. I was terrified! I ran upstairs crying 'I've had a shock, I've had a shock!' I was convinced I was going to die, there and then. I stood, panting melodramatically, waiting to die. But nothing happened. I can laugh at my terror now. But of course, electricity can injure if not treated with respect.

Diabetes is obviously rather more serious than a minor electric shock. But if you learn about the condition, what caused it, what is happening in your body, and, most importantly, how to look after yourself and keep fit, it need not be frightening. You can carry on doing the things you enjoy with very few limitations. If you ignore it and hope it will go away, it may cause you trouble.

This book is an introduction to diabetes – what it can feel like to have it and what the doctor may ask and may look for on examination. There is a section on the tests your doctor may do. A chapter discusses what you need to know straightaway and there is further information

1

to help as you continue in your diabetic career. Diet and other treatments for diabetes are detailed. The rest of the book is about keeping fit and enjoying life with diabetes.

The sequence in which this book is written is designed to be easy for someone with newly-diagnosed diabetes to follow. However, those of my readers who are experienced in diabetes may wish to go straight to the sections relating to enjoying life with diabetes (travel, sport and so on), specific aspects of treatment, self-monitoring or tissue damage. Each chapter can be read on its own.

I use proper medical terms throughout this book, always with explanations, so that you can interpret any 'Medspeak' you encounter in the surgery or clinic. There is also a glossary at the end. To enliven the book I have included stories about people with diabetes. These stories are based on real life but have been altered to protect the participants.

Throughout the book I have assumed that your doctor is male, your nurse and dietician female and so on. This is to save writing he/she throughout the book. But your doctor may be a woman – as I am – and indeed your nurse or dietician may be male. No offence is intended to those of the opposite sex.

This book is one doctor's description of some of the ways of assessing and helping people with diabetes. But there are many people with diabetes (over 98 million worldwide) and tens of thousands of doctors with a special interest in diabetes. The people who know most about *your* diabetes are you and the diabetes team who help you to care for it. It is to your own doctor that you must go for advice about your personal condition. If you have questions about what you have read in this book or about other aspects of your diabetes, please contact your diabetes team straightaway. Remember, diabetes care is a rapidly-moving field. Ask your diabetes team to help you to keep up-to-date with new ideas.

I could not have written this book without the support and encouragement of thousands of people with diabetes who have shared their experiences and their friendship with me over the years. One of them, who attended a British Diabetic Association/Outward Bound Course with a group of other people with diabetes said recently 'I feel more confident about being diabetic. It is not going to stop me doing anything in life I want to do. Being diabetic has made me a stronger person. I am happy and optimistic about my future as a diabetic.' Another said 'Diabetes isn't the problem people think it is. It's not the end. It's a beginning.'

1

SYMPTOMS OF DIABETES

Symptoms are unusual feelings or body changes you notice yourself. How do you know you have diabetes? What do you feel?

WHAT ARE THE SYMPTOMS OF DIABETES?

Nothing at all

Many people feel nothing at all. They go to a doctor for a routine check-up and are astonished to discover that there is glucose in their urine and, subsequently, to be told they have diabetes. 'But how can I be diabetic? I don't feel ill', they say. Some of you may look back and realise that you have, after all, been feeling below par. But some people are not aware of chemical imbalance in their bodies. Unfortunately, even though you do not feel unwell you must still take your diabetes seriously.

Thirst

Thirst or polydipsia (*poly* = much, *dipsia* = thirst) is a classic diabetes symptom. Your mouth may feel like the Sahara desert and many pints of fluid may fail to quench your thirst.

> Joe was 23 when he developed diabetes. In the week before it was diagnosed he would wake up and have a glass of water, then have three cups of tea for breakfast. He works hard on a building site and he would take two big bottles of Pepsi with him in the morning. But by lunchtime they were drunk and he had to buy other drinks from the corner shop – six little boxes of juice and four cans of shandy to

3

last the afternoon. At home he drank six or seven cups of tea and half a dozen beers, and still had to take a jug of water to bed with him for the night.

Not everyone is as thirsty as Joe, but many people get into the habit of having extra drinks at their breaks or mealtimes.

Polyuria

This means passing a lot of urine (*poly* = much, *uria* = urine). You may need to urinate often and pass big volumes each time. Where is it all coming from? Most people think it is because they are drinking so much. But it is the other way round. The high glucose levels in the blood of someone with diabetes spill over into the urine making it syrupy. This draws water out of the body producing large volumes of urine and making you thirsty.

Miss Green looked after her 84 year-old mother who was rather shaky and had had a weak bladder for some years. Her mother usually slept well but one night she woke up her daughter. 'I'm so sorry dear,' she said, 'I've wet the bed. I wanted to go so badly and I just couldn't get out to the toilet in time.' 'Never mind, mother,' said Miss Green, as she got a fresh sheet out of the cupboard. But this went on for several nights, so Miss Green called the doctor. Since her mother's diabetes has been treated there have been no more wet beds.

People do not usually have to keep getting out of bed to pass urine during the night but if you have diabetes the polyuria continues night and day. In frail, elderly people or in small children this can occasionally lead to bed-wetting. Polyuria is inconvenient for everyone – you learn where all the toilets are at tube stations and in shopping precincts.

Weight loss

Glucose, the simple form of sugar we can eat directly or derive from digesting sweet or starchy foods, is the body's main fuel. People with untreated diabetes cannot use this glucose properly. It overflows into the urine and is passed out of the body – wasted. So body tissues are broken down in an attempt to provide fuel for the body. Gradually you lose weight.

Doris, aged 56 years, had been feeling rather under the weather lately. She was thirsty, and it was irritating having to get up to the

4

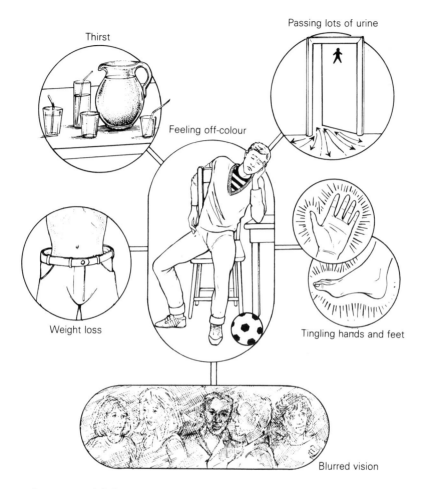

Thirst

Passing lots of urine

Feeling off-colour

Weight loss

Tingling hands and feet

Blurred vision

Symptoms of diabetes

toilet in the middle of the night. But she was eating well so there could not be much wrong. One weekend she decided to clear out her wardrobe. That blue suit, too tight for years, just try it once more before giving it to Oxfam. The suit fitted perfectly – in fact, it was a bit loose if anything. Doris was delighted. It was not until she went for her blood pressure check at her doctor's some months later

5

that she discovered she had lost some 20 pounds in weight over the past year. Then the doctor found her to have diabetes.

Diabetes is one of the causes of weight loss despite a good appetite. Some people actually have a craving for sugary foods.

Constipation

As you pass more and more urine, it becomes harder and harder to keep up with your fluid loss. Your body starts to dry out (become dehydrated). This can lead to constipation.

Tiredness, malaise, no energy

Malaise is uneasiness or a non-specific feeling that all is not well. Diabetes can make you feel tired and lacking in energy. You may feel that your get-up-and-go has gone. You may be so tired that you go straight to bed on your return from work.

Tingling

The chemical changes of diabetes can alter the function of the nerves, the cables that carry the electric signals between your brain and your body. This can produce tingling or pins and needles in hands or feet. These usually improve with treatment of the diabetes.

Infections

Mrs Bibi is 42 years old and works in the family greengrocer's shop. One evening, helping to unload the van, she scratched her foot on a crate of apples. She washed the wound but soon she forgot all about it as she hurried around the shop. Two days later her foot began to hurt. On inspection the wound was oozing pus and the foot was red and swollen. Her doctor said she had an infection and gave her antibiotics. But the infection was very slow to heal and further tests revealed diabetes. Once that was treated the foot infection healed.

All our body's defence mechanisms work best in a normal chemical environment. If the body's chemistry is awry, you may not be able to fight infection properly. In uncontrolled diabetes, the white blood cells which seek out and destroy bacteria, do not move as well as usual and the bacteria multiply.

Common infections in previously undiagnosed diabetics include boils or carbuncles, other abscesses, chest infections, urinary tract infections (e.g. cystitis) and thrush. Thrush can cause discharge, itching (pruritus) and soreness around the vagina in women (vulvitis or vaginitis) and the penis in men (balanitis). Once the diabetes is under control, antifungal cream will cure thrush. Any infection may be worse or take longer to resolve in people with high blood glucose levels due to diabetes.

Blurred vision

Just as stirring sugar into water makes it thick and syrupy, glucose in the blood alters its consistency. The body can equalize this to some extent but high glucose levels throughout can alter function of some body components. This includes the lens of the eye. Its focusing properties are disturbed and the vision may become blurred or hazy. Wait until your diabetes has been treated and your vision is stable before buying new glasses.

Austin was fed up with his glasses. He could not see the paper clearly and reading was a real strain. He clearly needed a new pair – something stronger. He went to an optician who gave him a new prescription. He chose some sophisticated new frames as well. It was very expensive but he was pleased with the result – for about two weeks. Then his vision changed again. His diabetes was diagnosed after an insurance medical check. Once it had been treated the blurring of vision settled and his old spectacles were fine. The optician would not take the new spectacles back.

THE PATTERN OF SYMPTOMS

How many symptoms?

Everyone is different. Do not expect to have all these symptoms. Some people have none of them. Usually thirst and polyuria occur together. Once your diabetes is treated your symptoms will settle.

How fast do the symptoms come on?

In younger people the symptoms may come on over days or weeks. They may be severe. It is usually very obvious that something is wrong. In older people the onset of diabetes can be very subtle. It may take weeks or months for anyone to realise that something is wrong. One man had had classic, albeit mild, symptoms of diabetes for 14 years before the diagnosis was made. But that is an exception.

SUMMARY

- A symptom is something unusual you notice about yourself.
- Symptoms of diabetes include thirst (polydipsia), polyuria, weight loss, constipation, infections which are severe or slow to resolve, tingling in the hands or feet and blurred vision.
- Some people have no symptoms at all.

2

THE DIAGNOSIS OF DIABETES

THE INITIAL CONTACT

There are many paths to the diagnosis of diabetes. Often the person who suspects that you may have diabetes is not the person who will care for your diabetes long-term. However, with the advent of increased health screening by general practitioners (GPs) in Britain it is becoming more likely to be your GP who finds that you are diabetic and who subsequently treats your diabetes in part or completely.

A routine check of a well person

Testing the urine for glucose forms part of most 'well man' or 'well woman' checks. Urine or blood glucose testing is also part of company or insurance medical tests. Most people with untreated diabetes will have glucose in their urine. (But not everyone with glucose in his or her urine has diabetes – see page 11.) Any doctor who does not usually care for your general health will almost certainly return you to your GP for further tests.

Going to your doctor because of symptoms of diabetes

If you have some of the symptoms described in Chapter 1, especially thirst and polyuria, your GP will probably check for diabetes. If he confirms the diagnosis he will then either refer you to a diabetes specialist clinic for further advice, or, if he has had training in diabetes care, will give you the help you need himself. Either way, he should give you some initial explanation about what diabetes is and how to start looking after yourself.

Going to a doctor for another reason

Some people discover they are diabetic because of the initial screening which doctors or hospitals perform in people who come to them for help with some other condition. I have seen people with diabetes who were initially referred as outpatients to urologists (specialists in urinary tract disease) with frequent urination, ophthalmologists (eye doctors) with blurred vision, dentists with dry mouths, dermatologists (skin doctors) with recurrent boils and so on. Patients may be admitted through casualty with severe infections and be found to have diabetes by the casualty officer. Sometimes people are first seen because of the tissue complications of diabetes (see chapter 12). The problem is that all the symptoms of diabetes bar the thirst and polyuria are non-specific and some are common. Most people who feel tired are not diabetic.

DIAGNOSING DIABETES

The point at which the diagnosis is confirmed varies. The formal diagnosis relies on one or more blood tests taken from a vein in your arm and tested by a laboratory. Until this has been done you do not know for certain that you have diabetes. Most doctors would not refer a patient to a diabetes specialist clinic until the diagnosis has been confirmed in this way.

Keeping the blood glucose normal

Normally, the blood maintains the blood glucose level at around 3.5 to 7.8 millimols (a unit of measurement) of glucose in every litre of blood. This is usually written as 3.5–7.8 mmol/l. For simplicity I will use 4–8 mmol/l in most of the book. In America, they measure the blood glucose concentration in milligrams per decilitre (mg/dl). 18 mg/dl equals 1 mmol/l and their normal range is about 60–140 mg/dl.

The body strives to maintain normality. If something goes wrong many mechanisms are brought into play to return everything to a normal state. This process is called homeostasis.

GLUCOSE IN THE URINE

The kidney filtering system is one of the ways in which the body attempts to maintain a normal blood glucose level. In most people the kidneys do not allow glucose to enter the urine if the blood concentration is below 8 mmol/l. If you have diabetes the blood glucose rises. The reasons for this are discussed in Chapter 4. As the glucose level rises above 8 mmol/l and then 10 mmol/l and upwards, glucose starts to leak into the urine. The blood glucose at which this occurs is called the kidney threshold or renal threshold (*renal* = kidney). This threshold is usually 10 mmol/l. The higher the blood glucose, the more glucose there is in the urine. On its way through the kidney filtering system this syrupy urine draws water with it.

Urine flows down the tubes draining the kidneys (called ureters) to collect in the bladder. When the bladder is full its walls stretch and you feel the desire to pass urine. The large volumes produced by someone with diabetes fill and stretch the bladder repeatedly.

You can already see that the concentration of glucose in the urine depends on many factors. At what point does the kidney begin to allow glucose into the urine? How much water is drawn in with the glucose? How long is the urine in the bladder before voiding? The amount of glucose filtered by the kidneys may fluctuate from hour to hour.

The kidney threshold for glucose

If someone has a low threshold for glucose, it will appear in the urine at a blood glucose concentration of, say, 6 mmol/l. This person is not diabetic but his or her urine will give a positive result on glucose testing. This condition is called renal glycosuria (*renal* = kidney, *glycos* = glucose, *uria* = in the urine). These people can be wrongly labelled as diabetic. This is one reason why it is essential to confirm the diagnosis of diabetes on blood testing.

If someone has a high threshold for glucose, say 16 mmol/l, their urine will be free from glucose until that level is reached. Thus, in them, a negative urine test does not mean that they are free from diabetes.

The blood glucose fluctuates all the time. Sometimes it may be above the renal threshold, sometimes below.

For all these reasons, urine testing may alert a doctor to the possible presence of diabetes, but it is not diagnostic. A negative urine test does not exclude diabetes.

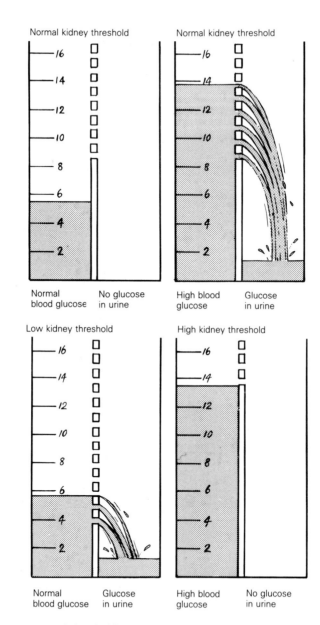

Differences in renal thresholds

GLUCOSE IN THE BLOOD

Having a blood test

Many people are frightened of having a blood test. Occasionally, the anxiety builds up out of all proportion to the very brief test. There is no need at all to be worried – the discomfort is akin to nicking yourself shaving or catching yourself on a rose thorn gardening. When you go to the surgery or hospital you will be asked to roll up your sleeve, and to sit down with your arm resting on a table. A band will be placed temporarily around your upper arm to make the veins stand up. Some people clean the skin with alcohol, some do not. The person taking the sample will hold your skin taut and slip the needle through the skin. It feels sharp or stings very briefly as it goes through the skin but in most cases that is all you will notice and within seconds the blood sample will be taken. You will be given a piece of cotton wool to press on the vein. Keep your arm straight and press firmly for one minute. (Bending the arm kinks the vein and can cause bruises.) And that is that. A few tips: keep really warm until just before the sample is taken (it makes your veins easier to find); relax as you sit down and do some deep breathing if you are nervous; concentrate on your summer holiday (if you relax it hurts less). If you are an experienced blood testee and have an especially good vein, show it to the person taking the sample.

What happens to your blood?

The sample will be put into a little bottle containing a chemical to preserve the glucose. The bottle is carefully labelled with your name, number (if in hospital) and the date. It is then sent to the laboratory with the accompanying request form from your doctor. (Do check the form when your doctor gives it to you. Make sure your name and other details are correct.) In the laboratory a receptionist checks in the sample and the request card and allocates it a laboratory test number. Then a technician puts the bottle into a centrifuge and spins it down to separate the blood cells from the fluid in which they float (plasma). The plasma is then put into the analyser (usually as part of an automatic line of samples) which measures the plasma glucose concentration. The result is then checked and printed or written onto a report form. The form will be sent to your doctor or his secretary. He must then extract your form from the heap of such forms he receives every day (in my own department this may be over a hundred forms a day) and match it with your records.

The plasma glucose concentration

Previously I have loosely referred to this as the blood glucose level. There are small differences between whole blood glucose concentrations and venous plasma glucose concentrations. There are also differences between glucose concentrations in a finger prick sample and one taken simultaneously from a vein.

Blood full of glucose and oxygen and other nutrients is delivered to parts of the body by arteries which divide into ever smaller branches. These branches eventually become capillaries which actually deliver the nutrients to the tissues. Waste substances are then drained from the tissues by small vessels which link up to form veins. Finger pricks obtain blood from capillaries. The tissues have used up some of the glucose by the time the blood reaches the vein.

Most laboratories measure venous plasma glucose and it is to this that I will be referring throughout this book when I talk about glucose levels taken from a vein and sent to the laboratory. Finger-prick testing measures capillary blood glucose.

The World Health Organisation criteria define three categories of plasma venous glucose concentration: normality, impaired glucose tolerance and diabetes. Obviously if you have had something to eat you will be absorbing glucose from digested food and your plasma glucose is likely to be higher than if you are starving. So it is important to know whether you are fasting (i.e. have had nothing to eat or drink except water for 14 hours) or whether it is a random blood sample.

Normal
- Fasting venous plasma glucose concentration below 7.8 mmol/l (140 mg/dl).
- Random venous plasma glucose concentration below 7.8 mmol/l (140 mg/dl).

Impaired glucose tolerance
- Fasting venous plasma glucose concentration below 7.8 mmol/l (140 mg/dl).
- Random venous plasma glucose concentration between 7.8 and 11.1 mmol/l (140–200 mg/dl).

Diabetes
- Fasting venous plasma glucose concentration above 7.8 mmol/l (140 mg/dl).
- Random venous plasma glucose concentration above 11.1 mmol/l (200 mg/dl).

In the presence of symptoms of diabetes, one fasting or one random blood test is sufficient to confirm the diagnosis. In the absence of symptoms, the diagnosis of diabetes can only be made on the basis of at least two separate confirmatory blood tests.

Impaired glucose tolerance

This is a grey area between absolute normality and definite diabetes. Some people with impaired glucose tolerance return to normal, some continue to have impaired glucose tolerance, some go on to develop diabetes. People with impaired glucose tolerance should follow a diabetic diet and keep themselves generally fit. They are at greater risk of heart trouble than people whose glucose is normal.

Glucose tolerance tests

In the old days, it was thought that diabetes could only be diagnosed by giving a standard dose of glucose and measuring the blood glucose levels before and at intervals thereafter. This is unnecessary in the majority of people. If you have diabetes it is usually obvious on two blood glucose tests. A few people with no symptoms of diabetes and inconclusive blood glucose tests may be offered an oral glucose tolerance test (OGTT). This involves swallowing 75 grammes of glucose in water and blood tests before and two hours afterwards. If the conditions of the test are not standardised it is possible to obtain three different results in the same person on three different occasions. You should have eaten your usual diet (i.e. with no restriction on sugary or starchy foods). You must sit still for the whole test and must not smoke.

WHAT NOW?

If you have been told that you have diabetes you should now possess the following information:

- A careful record of your diabetes symptoms (if any);
- One (symptoms present) or two (symptoms absent) venous plasma glucose concentrations written down in your own health record.

The next step is to find out who is going to assess you and your diabetes in general and who is going to care for you and your diabetes.

Every person with diabetes has the right to see a doctor with specialist training in diabetes. This doctor may be your own GP or one of his colleagues, but is more likely to be a hospital-based diabetes consultant working in a diabetic clinic. Unfortunately there are still some parts of Britain where such a specialist service is not readily accessible.

Either way, your GP will remain central in your health care, and it is very important that you discuss everything with him and keep him informed. Nowadays, most hospital diabetes clinics share diabetes supervision with the patient's GP – usually a very fruitful coalition for the patient.

SUMMARY

- There are many paths to the discovery of diabetes.
- Diabetes may be suspected when glucose is found in the urine, but this alone is not diagnostic. Some people without diabetes pass glucose in their urine. Some people with diabetes do not.
- The WHO criteria for diabetes are a fasting venous plasma glucose concentration above 7.8 mmol/l, or a random venous plasma glucose concentration above 11.1 mmol/l. Two such values are required to diagnose diabetes in someone with no symptoms of the condition.

3

ASSESSING A PERSON WITH DIABETES

Your doctor will want to listen to your story, ask some questions of his own and to examine you generally.

YOUR STORY

Tell the doctor exactly what you noticed wrong. Try to be specific about symptoms, if you can. It is often helpful to give the headlines first and then elaborate on them if necessary. Can you remember for how long the symptoms have troubled you? How bad are they? Are they interfering with your life? Have you had them before?

For example:

'Over the past two months I've been thirsty, drinking a lot of water and I keep passing urine. I've lost about a stone in weight.'

If your doctor asks for details you could say, 'I've got more and more thirsty over the past two months. Now I'm drinking about three big jugs of water a day and lots of tea. I get thirsty at night too. I'm going to the toilet every hour or two and I pass a lot of urine each time. I'm not sleeping very well because I have to get up to go to the toilet. Six months ago I used to weigh 11 stone and last night I only weighed 10 stone.'

But do not feel you have to have symptoms. Not everyone with diabetes does. It is also important to tell the doctor about any other symptoms you have, even if you do not think they are related to your diabetes. You might not think that easy bruising and thin skin could be related to diabetes. But it could if you were taking steroid tablets which had caused your diabetes and your easy bruising.

Who are you and what do you do? It helps your doctor to know what sort of person you are and what job you do. He may ask what the job involves – is it heavy work, or is your timetable very variable? Are you a shift or night worker? Do you have responsibility for other people's lives? Are you self-employed? Is your diabetes interfering with any aspect of your life?

Previous medical history

It is important that you tell any new doctor about your medical past. This includes major illnesses and any operation. Doctors usually ask about tuberculosis, rheumatic fever, epilepsy, kidney disease, heart trouble and high blood pressure. In someone with new diabetes it is also helpful to know about thyroid disorders and pernicious anaemia, other autoimmune disorders (see page 33), pancreatitis (see page 36) or pancreatic surgery.

Obstetric history

How many pregnancies have you had and how many babies? How much did your babies weigh? Diabetic women often have a history of big babies. Did you have diabetes or glucose intolerance in pregnancy?

Family history

Does anyone in your family have diabetes now, or did anyone that you know of in the past? Diabetes runs in families.

Drugs and allergies

By drugs I mean any medicine or remedy in any form – injections, pills, capsules, tablets, mixtures, elixirs, herbal extracts, vitamins, ointments, potions. It is very dangerous not to tell your doctor what you are taking as it may react adversely with something he gives you. Some drugs can cause diabetes or worsen it. These include steroids (e.g. prednisolone) and thiazide diuretics (such as bendrofluazide or Moduretic) which are used to treat high blood pressure or ankle swelling.

Some people, especially those from Asia, have a traditional doctor and a NHS doctor. Some traditional remedies may lower the blood glucose slightly – karela, for example. The problem with many herbal remedies is that they may contain toxic impurities and that the dose of any active ingredient is variable. Other people see homeopathic doctors or other alternative practitioners. You are, of course, entitled to seek whatever health care you wish, but it is not only courteous but safer to tell each practitioner that you are seeing the other(s).

If you have ever had an adverse reaction to any drug or medication it is vital that you tell every doctor you see about it. Such adverse reactions or allergies might include coming out in spots on taking penicillin, skin irritation caused by using sticking plaster or something more serious.

Eating and drinking

Your doctor may ask you about the sort of foods you usually eat, although he will probably leave detailed questioning to the dietician. Do you have religious or moral rules which preclude certain foods? It is also useful to know if you have to eat at unusual hours or cannot predict when you will eat.

Do you drink alcohol and if so, how much? Do you drink a lot of alcohol or have you ever drunk heavily in the past? It is important to be honest – large amounts of alcohol can damage the pancreas and cause diabetes, and other conditions for which it is important to be checked (see page 36).

Smoking

As smoking causes many different illnesses, any doctor will ask whether you smoke.

Your overall health

People who have a full medical examination for the first time are often mystified by the lists of questions that the doctor asks them. If you have gone to the doctor because you are passing a lot of urine, questions about chest pain and cough may appear to be straying from the point. But you may have symptoms which you have forgotten or which seem unimportant to you, but which can help the doctor to come to a diagnosis. However most people say 'No' to most of these 'screening' questions.

EXAMINATION

Most doctors will ask you to undress fully. Leave your underpants on unless asked specifically to remove these. Tell the doctor if your religion prevents you from revealing your legs or imposes other restrictions. Most surgeries and hospitals have women doctors who could examine you if you prefer, but you may have to wait for one to be found. Similarly, if you would prefer to see a male doctor, ask. Ask, too, if you wish a relative or friend to chaperone you. Doctors are trained to examine patients while standing on your right hand side and they will usually ask you to lie down on a couch so that they can examine you more readily. Do not be afraid to ask for help in undressing or getting on or off the couch – there will always be someone to help you. It is easier for the doctor to examine you if you are relaxed – although all doctors understand that you may not be feeling at all relaxed! Try taking calm, deep breaths and letting your muscles relax.

Signs of diabetes

General behaviour and appearance You may look outwardly normal and there may be no sign that you have diabetes. Other people with diabetes may be rather tired and perhaps irritable or listless. With very high blood glucose levels and severe chemical imbalance, you may be confused, semi-conscious or unconscious – but this is an uncommon finding in new diabetes.

If you have lost a lot of fluid you will be dehydrated. This can make your tongue dry and your skin may lose its usual elasticity. Many people with untreated diabetes lose weight and this may be obvious. A previously fit teenager can become very thin in a matter of weeks. You will all return to normal once your diabetes is treated. Some people may have white patches of pigment lack – vitiligo – a condition associated with autoimmune disorders, of which diabetes is one (see page 33). People who have an infection may be flushed or feverish and have a raised temperature.

You may have spots or boils on your face or elsewhere. Some people may notice fatty lumps on their upper eyelids by the nose (called xanthelasmata) or may have a white fatty ring around the coloured iris of the eye (called a corneal arcus). These may be signs that your cholesterol level is raised (see page 148). Some people have other skin problems with diabetes, which are discussed on page 123.

Heart and circulation Your pulse rate will probably be normal (about 60–90 beats per minute), although if you are anxious, infected, very dehydrated or in a state of severe chemical imbalance it may be fast. Your arteries (the blood vessels which carry oxygen and nutrient-rich blood from the heart to the tissues) may feel tortuous and wiggly if you have atherosclerosis or furring-up of the arteries (see pages 131, 141). Smoking is the commonest cause of this, but diabetes can cause it too. If the arteries are very furred-up the doctor will not be able to feel the pulses in your feet and legs. Sometimes it is possible to hear turbulent blood flow over areas of atherosclerosis by listening with a stethoscope in the neck or the groin, for example. This noise is called a bruit.

Your blood pressure may be normal, low or high. If you are dehydrated you may have a low blood pressure, which may fall further when you stand up. This is called postural hypotension. High blood pressure (hypertension) is more common in people with diabetes than in other people and may need treatment (see page 140). Some people with long-standing diabetes may have normal or high blood pressure sitting or lying down, which falls on standing (postural hypotension) because the nerves which control the blood vessels response to gravity have been damaged (see page 140).

Your heart will probably be of normal size and your heart sounds will probably be normal. If you have had untreated blood pressure for some time the heart may be enlarged because it has to pump more strongly to overcome the higher pressures in the arteries. Occasionally there may be murmurs (turbulent blood flow across the valves in the heart). These are usually of no major significance but may indicate that your largest artery, the aorta, has some atherosclerosis.

Your ankles may be puffy if your heart has been weakened – by a previous heart attack for example. But there are many causes of swollen ankles, the most common being standing up all day in hot weather.

Your lungs Your doctor will probably check that your breathing is normal. In people who are severely ill with new diabetes, there may be a very deep, sighing breathing, called Kussmaul breathing. This is to blow off acid from the body and is a sign that the person is very ill. The person's breath smells of acetone (pear drops or rotten apples).

Most people with diabetes have normal chest expansion and normally resonant lungs (checked by tapping the chest with a finger), and their breath sounds are normal. If you have a chest infection, there may be signs of this on examination, including a cough with green phlegm. Doctors call phlegm sputum.

21

Abdomen This is the area between the ribs and the groins. Most people call it their tummy or stomach, but strictly speaking the stomach is the bag inside on the left into which all your food is delivered when you swallow it. The abdomen can only be examined when you are lying flat and with your hands relaxed by your sides. If you tense your muscles the doctor will be unable to examine you. Occasionally the liver may be enlarged, this often settles with treatment. There may be tenderness over the bladder (in the lower abdomen) or kidneys (in your sides or loins) if you have a urinary tract or kidney infection.

If you have noticed itching, burning or discharge from the penis or the vagina, the doctor will examine these areas too and may take swabs to send to the laboratory. The swabs nearly always show *Candida albicans* – the thrush fungus which is easily treated.

The nervous system and senses This means the brain and the nerves which lead, like electric cables, to and from it. Most people with newly diagnosed diabetes will have no abnormal neurological (to do with the nervous system) signs. The detail in which the nervous system is assessed will depend, to some extent on your age and symptoms.

The eyes can be affected by diabetes in several ways (see page 24). The blurring of vision due to the changes in blood glucose concentration can reduce your visual acuity (i.e. the ease with which you can focus on the letters on the eye chart). This is usually temporary. Changes can occur in the back of the eye and the doctor will look at this with a magnifying torch called an ophthalmoscope. He may put drops in your eyes to make it easier to see the back of the eye.

The nerves which carry signals from the hands and feet to the brain can be affected by diabetes and this may mean that you have numb areas, especially on your feet, or have other changes in sensation (see page 139). Sometimes nerves which tell muscles what to do may be affected too.

After checking sensation and movement in face, arms and legs, your doctor will check your reflexes. These are found on both arms and legs, and your doctor will tap your elbows, wrists, knees and ankles with the tendon hammer to see if the muscles jerk reflexly. This shows that the nervous pathways are intact.

Feet Your feet are particularly vulnerable if you have diabetes. Your doctor will look at the shape of your feet and toes and deformities or unusual pressure areas. The skin is checked for injuries, ulcers, infection and general texture. He will feel the pulses on the top of the foot and behind the ankle. I have already discussed the need to check the sensation in the feet. Your doctor will notice your shoes as well.

Joints and ligaments These can be affected by diabetes long term, but it is unusual to see problems in a newly diagnosed diabetic.

All these findings will be noted down. Then the doctor summarises your problems. Here is an example of a case history as a doctor might write it down.

JOAN HOPKINS, AGE 42, HAIRDRESSER
Patient complains of:
– thirst
– polyuria
– 1 stone weight loss
– vaginal discharge

History of presenting complaint:
Well until two months ago
Gradual onset thirst (water by bed, carries drinks shopping)
Passes large volumes day/night = 10–12/2–3 times
11 stone in May 1989, now 10 stone
One week white vaginal discharge, severe itching and soreness

Previous medical history
No major illness
Varicose vein surgery 1984
Fractured right arm 1987

Obstetric history
Two pregnancies
Two children (Sarah 1978 birthweight 7 lbs; John 1980, 9 lbs)

Family history
Married, husband electrical fitter
Mother diabetic (on tablets), Father died stroke aged 69

Drugs
None

Allergies
None known

Diet
Vegetarian, but eats milk, cheese. Alcohol, 4–6 units a week.

Smoking
Stopped four years ago

Cardiovascular/respiratory systems
Dry cough following cold at present. Usually no symptoms

Gastrointestinal system
Weight falling
Appetite good, craves sugary foods
Slight constipation
No other symptoms

Genitourinary system
Urinary symptoms as above
Some burning on passing urine, no blood
Discharge and pruritus vulvae as above
Periods regular, LMP 10.2.92

Nervous system
Slight blurring of vision (one month)
No other symptoms

Endocrine system
No thyroid or adrenal symptoms

ON EXAMINATION
Tired, unwell
No anaemia, cyanosis (blueness), jaundice (yellowness)
No xanthelasmata or arcus
No lymph node enlargement
Normal breasts

Cardiovascular system
Pulse 84 beats/min, regular. Blood pressure 170/95 (lying and standing)
Carotid (neck artery) pulses normal, no bruits
Heart not enlarged

Heart sounds normal, no added sounds
No evidence cardiac failure
Peripheral pulses present, equal

Respiratory system
Respiratory rate 14/min
Expansion normal, equal
Percussion note resonant, equal
Breath sounds normal, no added sounds

Abdomen
Non-tender, no scars or masses
No enlargement liver, kidneys, spleen

Vaginal examination
Curd-like white discharge (swab sent), perineal redness, otherwise
examination normal

Nervous system
Eyes – visual acuity left 6/9, right 6/9
Lens normal
Fundi (the back of the eye) normal
Power and sensation normal, upper and lower limbs
Normal reflexes

Feet/legs
Blister right little toe (new shoes!)
Varicose vein surgery
Ingrowing toenail left great toe
Sensation and circulation normal

Diagnosis
Diabetes mellitus
Hypertension
Candida albicans
Blister and ingrowing toenail

The next stage would be some investigations.

TESTS

Blood glucose concentration

If the diagnosis has not been confirmed with a laboratory venous glucose sample, then it must be (see page 14).

If the diagnosis is known, the doctor may still want to check today's glucose level. Nowadays, many doctors do this with a desktop meter.

Glycosylated haemoglobin

This is a measure of long term glucose balance. Haemoglobin is the chemical which makes your red blood cells red. When the haemoglobin is being incorporated into the red cells glucose can bind with it. This process is called glycosylation. The more glucose there is in the circulation, the greater the proportion of haemoglobin that is glycosylated. This form of haemoglobin is called haemoglobin $A1_c$ and usually forms less than 8 per cent of the total haemoglobin (some laboratories have different normal ranges).

Other tests

A full blood count will check whether you are anaemic or have a raised white blood cell count which may indicate infection. Measurement of blood electrolyte level (see page 218) will indicate your body salt levels. Urea and creatinine assess state of hydration and kidney function (page 135). Cholesterol and triglyceride are blood fats which may be raised in untreated diabetes (page 148). A chest X-ray is done to exclude chest infections and look at the heart size. An electrocardiogram (page 130) checks the heart function. Microbiological examination of a midstream urine sample can show a urine infection.

SUMMARY

- Tell your doctor what (if anything) you have noticed wrong.
- Tell him your previous medical history, obstetric history and family history.
- Tell him what medication you take and whether you suffer from any allergies.

- Describe your eating habits and be honest about smoking and drinking alcohol.
- Your doctor will usually examine you carefully to check your general health and the effect (if any) that the diabetes has had upon it.
- Then he may do some tests including blood glucose level and haemoglobin A1.

4

WHAT IS DIABETES? WHY ME?

So now you know that you have diabetes and have had a careful initial assessment. But what is diabetes and why have you got it?

WHAT IS DIABETES?

Diabetes is a condition in which the blood glucose is above normal because your body can no longer use the glucose you absorb from digested food. The name was coined by Aretaeos the Cappedocian in the second to third century AD from a Greek word diabetes meaning siphon. 'Diabetes is a mysterious illness ... being a melting down of the flesh and limbs into urine.' Centuries later it was found that in some forms of diabetes the urine tasted sweet like honey (mellitus) and in others it was tasteless (insipidus). You have diabetes mellitus. Diabetes insipidus is due to lack of the water-concentrating hormone, anti-diuretic hormone, and is nothing to do with diabetes mellitus.

But it is very important to understand that the problem is not just one of blood glucose balance. Diabetes can affect many of the chemical processes and tissues in the body. It is a multi-system disorder. This is why your doctor and diabetes team check you over so carefully. Many people, even those who have had diabetes for years do not realise that diabetes care is not simply a matter of eating the proper diet and taking the diabetic tablets to correct the high blood glucose. For example, they do not connect their foot ulcer with having diabetes. But it is all part of the same condition. You and your doctors must care for your whole body not just your blood glucose.

So the true definition must be: diabetes mellitus is a chronic multi-system disorder defined by an abnormally high blood glucose concentration.

BODY GLUCOSE BALANCE

Food

We obtain glucose by digesting the carbohydrate foods we eat. These starchy or sugary foods (e.g. bread, potato, beans, rice, pasta, sugar, sweets, candy, biscuits) are first prepared by processing or cooking in an infinite variety of ways (for example, boiled potatoes, mashed

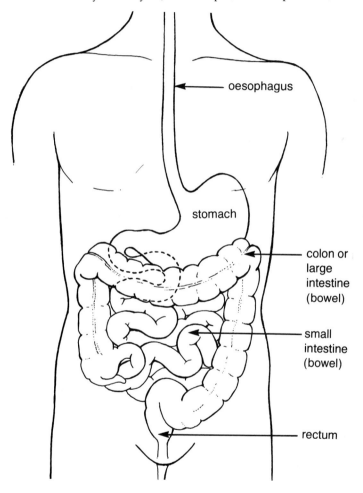

oesophagus

stomach

colon or large intestine (bowel)

small intestine (bowel)

rectum

The digestive system

potatoes, fried potatoes, chips, crisps etc.) Then we eat them. They are broken down into a lumpy mush by chewing and then swallowed. Already digestive enzymes (breakdown chemicals) in the saliva are starting to work on the food. The chewed mush passes down the gullet or oesophagus into the stomach (see page 29). There it is churned around and mixed with stomach juices which contain acid. This kills off most bacteria and helps to further break down the food. The stomach pushes the food out into the first part of the gut, the duodenum, where the digestive juices from the pancreas and the gall bladder (bile) are mixed in with the food. As it passes on through the duodenum into the jejunum and then the ileum, the food is being broken down into a thin soup containing simpler and simpler substances. As the soup of food and digestive juices pass through the small bowel (duodenum, jejunum and ileum) the simple particles into which the food has been digested are absorbed through the bowel wall into the bloodstream. This includes glucose which is the simple sugar into which most carbohydrate foods are broken down. Other simple sugars include lactose (from milk) and fructose (from fruit, although fruit sugar is also broken down into glucose). Undigested food, e.g. fibre, and other wastes are passed from the small bowel into the large bowel or colon and are eventually passed as faeces.

Glucose is the body's main fuel. As the glucose absorbed from the small bowel travels along in the bloodstream it first passes through the liver. The liver acts as a storage depot for glucose. Much of the glucose will stay in the liver until it is needed. But, without help, glucose cannot leave the bloodstream and enter the body cells (the tiny units from which all body tissues are made).

The chemical which allows glucose to enter liver cells and those of other tissues is called insulin. It is made in the pancreas in clusters of cells called the islets of Langerhans. These islets are dotted about the pancreas amongst the rest of the cells which are busy making digestive juices. Within the islets of Langerhans are the beta cells whose main job is to make insulin. You cannot see your pancreas, or feel it, for it lies hidden behind the stomach and in front of the backbone deep in your abdomen.

Insulin is a hormone, a chemical made in one group of cells and released into the bloodstream to influence processes elsewhere in the body. It is made inside the beta cell and stored as granules until it is needed. In a non-diabetic, a rising glucose triggers special nervous and chemical signals in the pancreas which stimulate the beta cells to release their stored insulin into the bloodstream. A falling glucose 'switches off' insulin release.

30

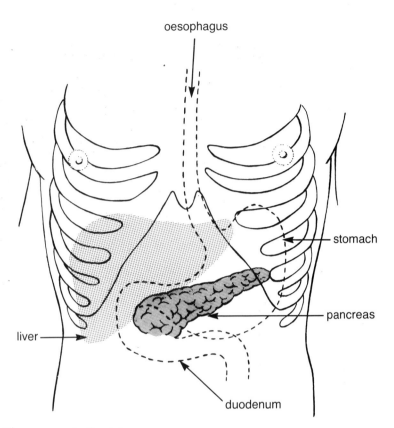

oesophagus

stomach

pancreas

liver

duodenum

The pancreas in the abdomen

The way in which insulin links with the body's cells and enables glucose to enter has been worked out in considerable detail by years of painstaking research all over the world. On the surface of many cells are specially-shaped areas called insulin receptors. They are shaped to be an exact fit for insulin, rather like a keyhole waiting for a particular key. The insulin acts as the key. When the insulin key fits into the keyhole, a chain of chemical changes occurs in the wall of that cell and glucose is passed through the cell wall, rather like a key opening a door.

So glucose cannot enter the body's cells without insulin, and insulin cannot work without insulin receptors.

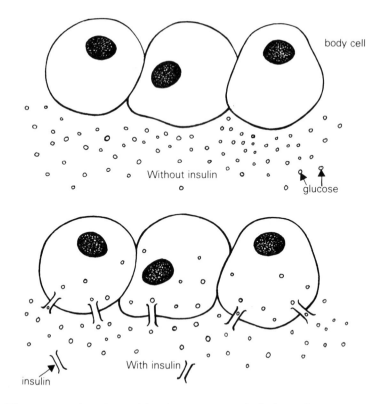

The presence of insulin enables glucose to enter the body's cells

Cells are like little factories – they have a considerable variety of functions. Once inside the cell, glucose is either burned up as a fuel or stored for future use. It is stored in big clumps called glycogen. When the blood glucose levels fall, as in vigorous exercise for example, the beta cells stop releasing insulin and the lack of insulin allows breakdown of glycogen back into glucose. This is either used up there and then or released into the bloodstream for other cells to use. The cells which use most glucose are muscles. It is glucose which fuels your press-ups or your walk to work. It is glucose which keeps your heart muscle pumping. But muscles can also use other fuels derived from fats. One part of the body is wholly dependent on glucose – the brain. It is glucose which keeps your brain ticking over and fuels those brilliant (and for that matter, not-so-brilliant) ideas.

Normally the body keeps all its body systems in balance and if any of its processes are upset it reacts to return them to normal (homeostasis – see page 10). Through its complex systems of insulin release and the storage of glucose or the breakdown of glycogen, the body maintains the blood glucose levels at about 4–8 mmol/l no matter what you do. A huge chocolate pudding or a 10 mile run cause no major fluctuation in blood glucose level. But if you have diabetes this finely tuned system fails. Two main factors appear to be involved – insulin manufacture and release, and insulin receptors.

TYPES OF DIABETES

Insulin-Dependent Diabetes Mellitus (IDDM)

This is the form of diabetes which predominantly affects children and young people. It is also called juvenile onset diabetes or Type I diabetes. This form of diabetes is due to a complete failure of insulin production.

People with IDDM appear to inherit a lack of protection from diabetes. Our genetic material is handed down to us in chromosomes which are double strands of a special protein called deoxyribonucleic acid or DNA for short. DNA is made of tiny particles called amino acids which are arranged in sequences. One of these amino acids (on Chromosome 6) is replaced with others in people with diabetes. One theory is that the person is then vulnerable to an upset, such as a viral infection, which can trigger the body to destroy its own beta cells. This process is called an autoimmune reaction (*auto* = self, *immune* = defence mechanism). It is really a natural example of chemical warfare, going on inside you. Foreign substances, called antigens, for example chemicals carried by bacteria, are detected by the body's defence cells – the white blood cells. They react by making antibodies which destroy the antigens. In diabetes, the white cells perceive substances on the wall of the beta cells as antigens and make antibodies which destroy them.

As the beta cells die, less and less insulin is made and released and the blood glucose rises rapidly. In IDDM, islet cells antibodies can be detected months or years before the development of diabetes, but when the major destructive process begins, it is rapid and most of the beta cells are destroyed within weeks. So other processes must be at work too.

People with IDDM are usually under 30 years of age, sometimes

33

children, who are slim (or even thin) and have had severe thirst, polyuria and weight loss for a few weeks. They usually feel ill. If they do not receive insulin quickly they will become extremely ill. Before the discovery of insulin in 1922, children with IDDM did not survive. But with insulin people feel better within days.

About one person in 400 has IDDM and the frequency is increasing.

Non Insulin-Dependent Diabetes Mellitus (NIDDM)

This form of diabetes is much more common than IDDM and tends to occur in the over 30s. Overall, one in 130 people have NIDDM and know it, another one in 100 have it without realising – a total frequency of about one in 60. Again, the frequency is increasing. However, the frequency of NIDDM varies among different communities. Known diabetes is about four times more common in the Asian community than in the rest of the population. Within the Asian community NIDDM starts in a younger age group (being most often diagnosed in the 30s or 40s) and the frequency increases with age so nearly one in five Asian people over 60 are known to have diabetes. This is an underestimate – the true frequency in some sections of the Asian community can be as high as 25 per cent. Diabetes is also more common in people whose ancestors came from Africa or the Caribbean Islands.

There is some debate as to the exact cause of the problem. Once again the vulnerability to diabetes is inherited – more strongly than in IDDM. Indeed, it has been estimated that as many as 25 per cent of the first degree relatives (that is parents, brothers, sisters) of someone with NIDDM had, have or will develop diabetes. People with NIDDM are capable of making insulin – indeed for years it has been thought that they may even make more than non-diabetic people. However, recent work has shown that older ways of measuring insulin measure insulin-related chemicals as well as insulin, producing falsely high 'insulin' levels.

There are several theories. One is that NIDDM is due to a lack of insulin receptors or abnormalities within the receptor. Overweight people have been shown to have fewer insulin receptors and it was thought that such people would have to make more insulin to try to overcome this problem. Eventually, the exhausted beta cells 'wear themselves out'. High plasma insulin levels have been found in overweight people with NIDDM. Another theory is that the beta cells are making some insulin, but not enough and they are not releasing it at

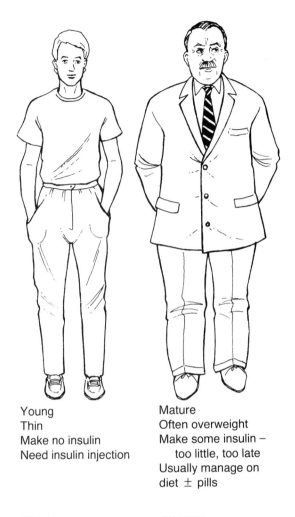

Young	Mature
Thin	Often overweight
Make no insulin	Make some insulin –
Need insulin injection	too little, too late
	Usually manage on
	diet ± pills

IDDM   *NIDDM*

the right time. This can be demonstrated by giving people a glucose meal or injecting sterile glucose into a vein and measuring the insulin response.

There has been much excitement by the discovery that in people with NIDDM the beta cells are replaced with a solid, stranded material called amyloid. An apparent amyloid precursor has been found in beta cells, and in the bloodstream. But, as yet, there is no proof that this is the cause of diabetes rather than the end result of a destructive process.

It seems likely that several factors may combine to produce the same end result – an inability to cope with glucose. Overweight people do usually need more insulin per unit body weight (e.g. a unit of insulin per kilogram of body weight per 24 hours) to return their glucose to normal than a slim person (e.g. a third of a unit of insulin per kilogram per 24 hours). This is probably a cause of diabetes in some instances.

Other causes of diabetes

Pregnancy Diabetes or glucose intolerance can occur during pregnancy because of the dramatic rises in sex hormones at that time. This is called gestational diabetes. It may disappear completely after your baby is born, but can continue long term. If you have had gestational diabetes in one pregnancy you are likely to have it again in later pregnancies. And you are more likely than other women to become diabetic later on so you should maintain a normal weight, exercise regularly and keep an annual check on your blood glucose.

Pancreatic damage or surgery If you have had inflammation of the pancreas, the most common cause of which is long term alcohol excess, or an operation on the pancreas, the beta cells may be removed or damaged and you may develop diabetes. In addition, the cells which make pancreatic digestive juices may also be damaged and you may not digest your food properly. Weight loss and fatty, pale faeces, should alert you and your doctor to the need to add pancreatic extracts to your food or to swallow them as capsules. People who have drunk this much alcohol may have heart damage, brain damage and nerve damage. There are other causes of pancreatic inflammation too.

Drugs – steroids, other hormones, and thiazides Steroids are the hormones (see page 30) made by the adrenal glands which sit on top of the kidneys. In the small quantities usually produced in the body, they are essential for our survival. However, they are also useful in treating allergic conditions, like asthma, and severe inflammation like some forms of muscle problem or artery inflammation. In these big doses, they can cause diabetes. The more steroids you have to take, the higher the blood glucose. When the dose falls, so will the glucose, but you may remain diabetic.

The sex hormones in the contraceptive pill can cause glucose intolerance, or worsen existing diabetes.

Thiazide diuretics are pills given to increase urine production in conditions like high blood pressure and heart failure with swollen ankles. If you have any tendency to diabetes, thiazides may bring it out into the open.

Other hormone conditions Thyroid hormone overactivity (thyrotoxicosis) or growth hormone overactivity (acromegaly) can be associated with diabetes. Overproduction of steroid hormones by the body can also cause diabetes.

Iron deposition Iron deposition in the pancreas can cause diabetes. This occurs in people on treatment for thalassaemia (an inherited blood condition) and in haemochromatosis.

Tropical diabetes This does not occur in Britain. It is seen in tropical countries and is thought to be related to starvation or perhaps to contaminants in food.

WHY ME?

Some of you will have been able to identify the type of diabetes you have, but many may still be unsure. Do not worry, it is not essential to label your diabetes as the treatment will simply be tailored to you and your needs.

Some of you may be teetotal men or women on no medication with no family history of diabetes. You may not be able to find anything to blame for your diabetes – in your case it has just happened. Although it is human nature to look for an event or person to blame when we become ill, it is not always a good idea to do this as it can lead to frustration and retrospection when one should be looking ahead to feeling better and getting on with life.

SUMMARY

- The two main types of diabetes are IDDM and NIDDM diabetes.
- IDDM occurs mainly in thin under 30s with rapid onset of

severe symptoms. It requires insulin treatment. It is caused by insulin deficiency.

- NIDDM occurs mainly in overweight over 30s with more gradual onset of variable symptoms. It can usually be treated by diet alone or diet and pills. It is caused by a combination of inadequate insulin release and insulin resistance.
- Other causes of diabetes include pregnancy, pancreatic damage, steroids, thiazides and other drugs.
- Whatever its cause diabetes can always be treated.

5

GETTING STARTED

The doctor has told you that you definitely have diabetes. You may have been expecting it, or it may have come as a shock. Until they are told that the diagnosis is certain most people have been hoping that it is all a mistake. 'This can't be happening to me.' It can be especially startling for people who have had no symptoms of diabetes. 'How can I be ill if I don't feel ill?'

COMING TO TERMS WITH DIABETES

All of us think that our bodies should work perfectly. Illness is what happens to other people. When you become ill, especially when you develop a long-term illness, you react in different ways. Some people think it must be someone's fault. You look for someone, or something to blame. 'If my wife hadn't left me I would never have got diabetes.' 'It's all because that man drove into my car. It was the shock that did it. He gave me diabetes.' But as the previous chapter shows, most people who have diabetes are born with the potential to develop the condition.

Other people think it is all their own fault. 'I must have done something wrong.' 'I ate too much sugar.' You perhaps feel that you are being punished. 'God is punishing me because I have done something wrong. He is trying me.' But it is not your fault that you have diabetes. Nor is it anyone else's fault.

For some, the discovery of diabetes is a numbing blow and you feel as if your world has come to an end. Everything seems impossible, your plans are shattered, and there is no hope. Some people favour the ostrich approach. 'If I don't think about it, it will go away.' 'It isn't really happening. It is all a dream.' But if you bury your diabetes in the sand, you will get sandy too.

There are people who are very matter-of-fact about their diabetes. You will betray little emotion about it all and carry on at work and at home as if nothing has happened. Some people are good at coping with new problems in this way. Others find themselves reacting with anger or sorrow later.

Most people with newly-diagnosed diabetes have a mixture of emotions. Shock; some anger at fate for giving you this; some tears that you are not as well as you thought you were; some pretending it is not happening. But most people cope admirably with their new condition.

No-one comes to terms with diabetes overnight. But, gradually, try to accept that you have a condition which will, in the majority of cases, be with you for ever. It will need some attention from you every day. This may just be in terms of watching what you eat and checking your blood glucose occasionally, or it may be managing your insulin injection treatment. You will need regular medical check-ups – at least once a year. Your diabetes can make you unwell in years to come, but this is less likely if you look after yourself now, and continue to do so.

Do not be too tough on yourself. There is no right or wrong way to come to terms with having diabetes. It is not wrong to shout or cry or bottle it up. Learn about your condition and its management step by step. No one is ever a perfect diabetic. After all, no one is ever a perfect human being!

Fears and worries

Most people know very little about diabetes until it happens to them or to one of their family. They just hear about the dramatic aspects and the old wives' tales. So let me put some of these stories right straightaway.

Diabetes rarely makes people collapse dramatically, as portrayed in television dramas. Diabetes does not make people go mad. Diabetes will not stop you from having a family. Diabetes will not stop you from being a good mother, father, wife, husband. Diabetes rarely interferes with people's jobs. Diabetes will not make you go blind if you look after yourself. Diabetes will not stop you from enjoying your food. Diabetes will not stop you from having fun.

Think positively

Some people feel that becoming diabetic, despite its demands on their body and their time, actually enriches their life. A young woman who had recently developed diabetes said 'Being diabetic has made me a stronger person.' Another, who had changed from an overweight, inactive person eating junk food to a slim man who ate healthy food and exercised regularly said 'I'm fitter now than I've ever been.'

THE FIRST FEW DAYS

Information you need from your doctor

The diagnosis You need to know that you definitely have diabetes. Ask your doctor to tell you the diagnostic blood glucose values.

The cause Has the diabetes arisen because of an inherited tendency to diabetes? Is it secondary to another condition or being worsened by another condition which needs separate treatment? If so, what is it and what treatment does it require?

If you are taking medication which has precipitated your diabetes (e.g. steroid pills) or which is worsening it (e.g. thiazides – water or blood pressure pills) you need to know this. Should you stop this medication, reduce the dose or change it to something else? It can be dangerous to stop steroid pills suddenly.

Chemical imbalance Is your problem mainly the glucose imbalance of your new diabetes or are other body chemicals awry? Does any of the chemical imbalance need urgent treatment? If so, what?

Tissue damage Has your diabetes damaged any of your body tissues? If yes, which tissue and what treatment is needed? Is the treatment urgent?

Diet

The foundation of diabetes treatment is sensible eating. The right foods in the right quantities at the right times. But don't panic. If you eat the wrong thing nothing terrible will happen. Eventually you will be able to tailor the rest of your diabetes treatment to the healthy eating pattern which suits you best.

What to eat and drink If you eat or drink a glass of cola or some boiled sweets, the glucose they contain enters the bloodstream rapidly and your blood glucose rises fast. But your body cannot cope with glucose

41

as well as other people's. So you will not clear all this glucose. Your blood glucose will remain high for some time. If, on the other hand, you eat starchy, high fibre carbohydrate foods like beans or wholemeal bread, they are digested slowly and the glucose that they contain arrives in the bloodstream slowly so that your body has a chance to deal with it. So cut down on sugar and sugary foods.

Your body is not very good at coping with fat, either. Your blood fats may be high (see page 148). So it is sensible to eat less fat. Cut the fat off your meat and be sparing with butter and greasy foods.

Quench your thirst with a variety of drinks – water, tea, coffee or sugar-free 'diet' drinks. Do not drink colas and other fizzy drinks that contain glucose or sugar (sucrose). Avoid alcohol at present – you can drink alcohol in moderation when your diabetes is sorted out.

How much to eat If you are thin obey your appetite. If you feel hungry eat. If you are overweight you must watch the amounts you eat. Cutting out sugar and reducing fat will help you to lose weight but you should also watch the total quantities that you eat. Try to take smaller helpings. You may need to eat less than your appetite demands. Fill the gaps with vegetables – lettuce, cabbage, celery, tomato etc.

When to eat Eat three meals a day, spaced out evenly. If you are on insulin treatment, eat three snacks a day as well – mid-morning, mid-afternoon and before bed.

Diet alone An adjustment to your diet may be all you need to control your diabetes. In this case it is very important that you stick to it. After all, no one wants to take tablets or injections unless they are strictly necessary.

Pills

Your doctor may prescribe pills (see Chapter 8) to help your pancreas to release more insulin and to help the insulin to work more efficiently in the body tissues. These pills are called oral hypoglycaemic drugs (*oral* = taken by mouth, *hypo* = low, *glycaemic* = blood glucose). Ask the name of your pills. Write it down. Make sure you know exactly what dose to take and at which times of day.

Most glucose lowering drugs carry the risk of lowering the blood glucose below normal – that is below 4 mmol/l. If this happens you may notice unusual feelings or become unwell (see page 101). It is called hypoglycaemia. The symptoms include confusion, slow thinking, sweating, shaking and palpitations (a fast heartbeat). If you feel like this eat some glucose or sugar and contact your doctor or diabetic sister when you feel better.

Insulin

If you are not making any insulin you will need insulin injections to replace the missing insulin. This is nothing to be frightened about. The injections are given through special, very fine needles which sting no more than a gnat bite when they go into the skin. Soon, you will learn how to give the injections yourself and it will become as routine as styling your hair or shaving. Chapter 9 describes insulin treatment in detail.

Today you need to know the name of your insulin, the dose your doctor advises and when to take it – usually about 20 minutes before breakfast and 20 minutes before your main evening meal. Write this information down.

The doctor, diabetes sister or other diabetes team member will show you how to draw up your insulin (or set your insulin pen) and how to inject. Often people give their own first injection and continue to give their own insulin. It is not nearly such a big hurdle as most people imagine. You just pinch up a fold of skin and fat, put the needle in, push the plunger down, pull the needle out and press on the injection site briefly. It can take less time to do than reading the last sentence aloud.

Insulin can cause hypoglycaemia. If you feel muddled, slow thinking, sweaty, shaky or have palpitations, eat some glucose or sugar and then call your diabetes adviser.

Diabetes card

Your diabetes adviser will give you a card to carry on you all the time. It is important that you carry it. If you have an accident or become ill and have to go to hospital, the doctors need to know that you have diabetes.

Carry glucose

If you are on glucose-lowering pills or insulin injections you must carry glucose tablets (e.g. Dextrosol, Lucozade, Boots etc.) or sugar on you all the time just in case you become hypoglycaemic.

Hypoglycaemia is usually easy to cope with, but it is important to be prepared.

Checking your own blood glucose

You need some means of monitoring your own condition so that you can see if your diet and any other diabetes treatment is working. At one time everyone with diabetes tested their urine for glucose either by dropping urine and water onto fizzy tablets, or by dipping a strip into the urine. Nowadays, people with all types of diabetes are monitoring their own blood glucose directly. You do not have to do this at the beginning but most people find that self-monitoring of blood glucose gives them a lot more confidence in looking after their diabetes.

Your diabetes adviser will help you to learn how to monitor your own blood glucose (see also Chapter 6). It is well worth it.

Work

In most instances, you will not need time off work. However, if you are feeling unwell or if you are starting insulin treatment, it is sensible to take a few days off work until your diabetes is sorted out and you are feeling better.

A few people taking insulin (and sometimes glucose-lowering pills) will need to review their job. Airline pilots, drivers of passenger carrying vehicles or large goods vehicles, operational firemen, divers and those in some other high risk occupations will probably not be allowed to continue in their current post. Discuss this with your doctor and your employer, the situation is changing (see page 154).

Driving

The British Driving Licence which many of you will be carrying states 'You are required to tell the Drivers Medical Branch, DVLC, Swansea, SA99 1TU at once if you have any disability (includes any physical or mental condition which affects (or may in future affect) your fitness as a driver if you expect it to last more than 3 months.' Diabetes is such a condition and you are compelled by law to inform the DVLC (now called DVLA) as soon as it has been diagnosed. The new licence mentions diabetes specifically. There are similar requirements in other countries. (See pages 154 and 157).

Motor insurance companies regard diabetes as a 'material fact'. In other words you are strongly advised to tell your car insurance company that you have diabetes.

Do not drive a car, or ride a bicycle or motor bike for a week after starting glucose-lowering pills or insulin injections – discuss the exact length of time with your diabetes adviser.

Back-up

All over the world there are groups of people with diabetes who are willing to befriend new diabetics and help them to learn how to manage their condition. The British Diabetic Association (BDA) is one of the oldest of these organisations and there are local BDA groups throughout the country. Ask your diabetes adviser for the name and address of your nearest BDA group. Join your local diabetes association – it will provide information and support.

Help

Very important Before you leave the clinic, surgery, or hospital, make certain that you have written down the name(s) and telephone numbers of the people to contact if you are in difficulties with your diabetes. This includes an out-of-hours contact number. If things do go wrong one can almost guarantee that it will be at 3 am on a Bank Holiday.

If you need help telephone sooner rather than later. The father of one of my patients with diabetes always taught his son that 'No question is ever stupid if it has to be a question'. All health care professionals would rather answer a simple question now than have to give you emergency treatment later. Many people are worried about troubling their GP and even more worried about troubling hospital staff. Diabetes is a condition in which there is constant personal contact between patients and staff at all levels. Much of the day-to-day contact is by telephone. So you need never be afraid to bother the doctor or the rest of the diabetes team – that is what we are there for.

SUMMARY

- Learn to live with your diabetes.
- Make sure you write down the information you need to keep you going for the first few days – what is going on; what tests or changes in existing treatment are needed; what to eat; what pills

or insulin to take; how to check your glucose; what to do about work.

- Carry a diabetic card and emergency glucose or sugar.
- Tell the DVLA and your motor insurance company you have diabetes.
- Join your local diabetes association.
- Make sure you know who to call for help. Write down their telephone number.
- Do not be afraid to ask for help. That is what we are here for.

6

BLOOD OR URINE GLUCOSE TESTING

This is the key to freedom. If you can know, with certainty, what your blood glucose is at any time, anywhere, then you can adjust your own treatment.

Technology is moving very fast. By the time this book is published there will be newer testing techniques. All the current tests rely on obtaining a drop of blood from a finger tip or ear lobe and placing it on a strip which either changes colour or transmits signals directly to a meter. The colour changes can be read by eye or by a meter.

THE LABORATORY IN YOUR HAND

We believe laboratory results because we know that tests are done carefully, with trained precision and quality assurance on well-maintained equipment. If you are to produce similarly accurate results, you too must perform the test carefully, with trained precision on well-maintained equipment. If you do not follow the instructions exactly, literally down to the last second, the results you obtain will be at best meaningless, at worst disastrous.

But these tests are simple and, with practice, you will have no difficulty in obtaining results comparable with those of a big laboratory.

Preparing your fingers

Most people use their fingers although a few use their ear lobe while looking in a mirror. Your hands should be clean – wash them in warm

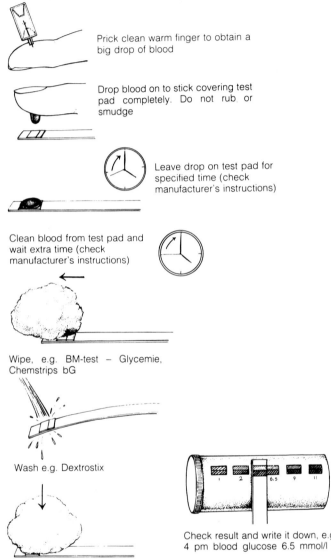

Prick clean warm finger to obtain a big drop of blood

Drop blood on to stick covering test pad completely. Do not rub or smudge

Leave drop on test pad for specified time (check manufacturer's instructions)

Clean blood from test pad and wait extra time (check manufacturer's instructions)

Wipe, e.g. BM-test – Glycemie, Chemstrips bG

Wash e.g. Dextrostix

Blot e.g. Glucostix. Visidex

Check result and write it down, e.g. 4 pm blood glucose 6.5 mmol/l

Measuring blood glucose

48

water, rinse all soap off and dry them on a clean towel. There is no
need to use antiseptic swabs – they make your result inaccurate. If
your hand is warm nothing else need be done. If you have difficulty
getting blood out or it is cold, try to warm your hand up. Also hold it
downwards towards your legs and shake the hand vigorously. You
will see the fingertips go pink with blood.

Pricking your fingers

You can simply use a sterile lancet (they are manufactured for single
use only). Most people find an automatic finger-pricker helpful. These
devices include Autoclix, Autolet II, Monojector, Penlet, Soft-touch
and others. Load the lancet into the device and then press a platform
onto the side of your finger. To start with you may find it easier to rest
your hand on a table. Then trigger the device. If you are the only
person using the finger-pricker you can reuse platforms if they are
clean. If someone else uses the device they must have a new platform
as well as a new lancet – and so must you when you next use it. There
are usually several different platforms for different pricking depths so
find the one that suits your fingers.

If your finger is warm the blood will ooze out on its own. If not,
milk it up from the base of the finger. Do not squeeze the finger-tip
tightly as this dilutes the blood with fluid and gives you sore fingers.

MEASURING THE BLOOD GLUCOSE CONCENTRATION

Colour-change strips

The first testing system was Dextrostix from which the blood had to be
washed before reading. These are rarely used today. The two largest
manufacturers of colour change strips are BM which produce BM
glycemie strips 1–44 (Chemstrips bG in USA) read by Reflolux meters,
and Ames which produce Glucostix read by Glucometers. There are
others including Hypoguard GA.

Before starting you should have checked that the strips are in date.
Hold the strip with the reagent pad upwards and drop the blood onto
the pad, covering it. Just enough, not too much and not too little, with
no smears. Instantly start timing with a watch with a second hand.
The glucose in the blood is reacting with the glucose oxidase in the
pad to produce a colour change in the dyes with which the pad is

impregnated. As soon as the time indicated in the instructions is up, wipe the blood off firmly with cotton wool (BM strips) or blot it off firmly (Glucostix). Wait the remaining time and match the colour with the range on the bottle from which you took the strip. Use a good light, and keep out of the rain or wind while doing the test.

If you are using a meter, follow the instructions in every detail. This always includes first calibrating the meter for that bottle of strips. When you take the strip out check the visual reading with that on the meter. If they are different do the whole test again. The most likely reason for problems are smeared or incompletely covered strips.

Biosensors

This exciting new technology has revolutionised home monitoring. The glucose sensor is available as a pen or a credit card shape. The test strips are individually foil-wrapped and are inserted into the sensor before you prick your finger. The test strip contains a glucose oxidase coated pad. Press the button as soon as the blood is placed on the pad. The reaction generates a tiny electric current which is sensed by the meter. In 30 seconds the result can be seen on a digital liquid crystal display. Exactech is the most widely used.

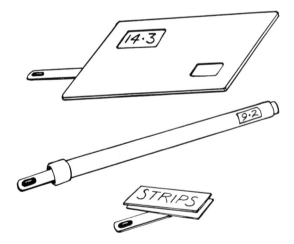

Glucose biosensors

50

As with meters it is essential that the biosensor is calibrated for each new pack of strips. The lack of visual confirmation (no colour change to read) is a drawback. If you do not do the test properly you have no way of realising that the result is inaccurate. As with other strips, cold wind or rain will obviously affect the result and it under-reads at low temperatures. Check that the strips are in date. This device is extremely accurate when used properly.

How do you get blood testing equipment?

All these devices should be obtained via your diabetes adviser. If you have no-one to advise you buy one from a pharmacist or medical shop. However, if possible get an expert to show you how to use it. In Britain, lancets and test strips are available on GP prescription. Meters are provided in various ways, depending on your diabetes service. At the time of writing patients have to buy the ExacTech biosensor but the strips are prescribable.

When to test

Whenever you want to or need to. If you are worried about your glucose, check it. Routinely you should check at least once a day. If you are a new diabetic, have changed your treatment, are pregnant or feel unwell, you must check your glucose four times a day. The standard times are before each meal and before bed. Pregnant women may be asked to check some after-meal (post-prandial) levels as well. If you are taking glucose-lowering pills, it is usually sufficient just to test before breakfast, fasting. On any treatment, if your blood glucose is above 19 mmol/l (342 mg/dl) and you feel ill, check every 2–4 hours.

Recording the result

Some meters (Glucometer M, Reflolux M) have memories which will record a specific number of glucose tests. There are also systems in which the meter can download directly into a computer. However, most patients still write down their results in diaries. These results are your record, not the clinic's, although it helps if your doctor and/or diabetes adviser go through the results with you. There is no point in writing down imaginary results. Who are you fooling? Yourself. Most doctors can spot an invented record, even if they say nothing. If you have done no tests, say so.

It is important to be able to spot trends, so write the results in columns with the time of day at the top. The figure shows a page from a busy young woman's record. Scattered numbers in your appointment diary are helpful at the time but hard to evaluate later.

PROBLEMS

Poor vision

If you cannot see at all, there are talking meters – ask your diabetes adviser or your diabetic association. If you can see a little but not well enough to match colours, the Exactech Companion has a large number display – ask to see one. If you have diabetic eye disease your colour vision may not be optimal. Use a meter or biosensor. People who know they are colour blind should do this.

Carelessness

Most problems are due to failure to follow the instructions for the strips or meter. Overfamiliarity breeds contempt. If you do not time the reaction properly you will get nonsense results. If you wipe the blood off on your trousers (I have seen it done) you will get very dirty trousers, and a dubious result. Get a proper sample and do not smear the blood. Keep the strips dry and in date.

Sticky finger

If you have anything sweet on your fingers all the test strip will measure is your finger candy level. This is a common trap in people with hypoglycaemia who have been eating glucose tablets. They get a high reading, think they are better, then become hypoglycaemic again.

The aim

You are aiming for a blood glucose concentration between 4 and 8 mmol/l (72 and 144 mg/dl). Below 4 mmol/l is heading for hypoglycaemia. Above 10 mmol/l (180 mg/dl) is too high and, if such high levels persist, may make you feel unwell, in addition to putting you at risk of tissue damage. It takes a lot of hard work to keep the blood glucose between 4 and 8 mmol/l. So do not get upset by the occasional value over 10 mmol/l. If you are taking glucose-lowering pills or insulin, you should go to bed with a blood glucose of 6 mmol/l or more (108 mg/dl) to protect you from night-time hypoglycaemia. Before breakfast you should aim for a fasting blood glucose between 4 and 6 mmol/l (72 and 108 mg/dl).

October '90.

Date	7.00	11.45	6.30	10.00	Comments
15th Mon	7	12	4	9	Blood Finished
16th Tues	11	6	9	6	Driving test - failed
17th Wed	6	9	6	8	
18th Thur	6	4	2	6	Had flu vaccine
19th Fri	12	18	10	10	
20th Sat	18	17	20	13	
21st Sun	16	12	22	18	increased Ultratard 38u

October '90.

Date	7.00	11.45	6.30	10.00	Comments
22nd Mon	16	17	9	20	
23rd Tues	10	9	18	17	
24th Wed	16	12	18	15	
25th Thur	10	10	20	11	
26th Fri	18	12	11	20	increased Eve Actrapid
27th Sat	12	16	13	11	
28th Sun	10	9	12	20	

Dosage
Actrapid 14 units, 6 Evening
Ultratard 38 units

Blood glucose diary

53

URINE GLUCOSE TESTING

This is an indirect method of estimating the blood glucose and its limitations are discussed on page 11. However, many people still use it and some doctors advise urine testing for most non-insulin-treated patients. Ensure that your strips are in date and dry. Hold the strip into the stream of urine, tap off the excess liquid and start timing it. Glucose oxidase in the pad reacts with glucose and the dye in the pad to produce a colour change. When the time is up match the colour against the chart on the bottle. If you prefer, pass urine into a completely clean container and dip the strip in. Then proceed as above.

It helps if you and your diabetes adviser check your renal threshold (page 11) before you use urine testing. You can do this by collecting urine for known time periods and matching urine glucose with simultaneous blood glucose samples. If you lose glucose into the urine very easily, or with difficulty, urine testing is not helpful in monitoring your diabetes.

Do the urine tests at the same intervals as blood tests, but remember that the urine reflects an average of the ups and downs of blood glucose over the time it has been filtered through the kidneys and collected in the bladder.

The aim

You are aiming to have no glucose in the urine. The old counsel of keeping a touch of sugar in the urine may lead to persistently high blood glucose levels as most people have a renal threshold around 10 mmol/l (180 mg/dl).

SUMMARY

- Blood glucose testing is the key to freedom for people with diabetes.
- Choose the method which suits you and use it carefully.
- Test regularly to keep a check of your diabetes, and at other times when you are worried or ill, or you are doing something unusual.
- Write the results down in a way that is easy to read.
- Act on abnormal results.
- Use urine testing if you prefer or if you cannot do blood tests, but be aware of its limitations.

7

DIET

The dictionary defines a diet as 'a mode of living, now only with especial reference to food'. This emphasises the integral part that eating plays in our lifestyle. Food is our means of staying alive, our comfort, a way of sharing or giving, our responsibility to our families and a great pleasure. The diet you need for your diabetes is still all of these things. In fact, it is the diet we should all be eating. In general, people with diabetes eat a much healthier diet than the rest of the population.

There are two parts to your diabetic diet. What you eat and drink and how much you eat and drink. It does not need to be complicated. You do not need to weigh out every morsel of food. You do not have to calculate complex exchanges, although some people on insulin injection treatment find these helpful. Nothing terrible will happen if you make the occasional mistake.

WHAT YOU EAT

Food is made up of carbohydrates, proteins, fats, fibre, minerals, vitamins and water. Carbohydrates, proteins and fats can be used by the body as fuels, for growth or for storage. Their fuel potential is measured in calories or kilojoules (one calorie = 4.2 kilojoules). Fats contain twice as many calories, weight for weight, as carbohydrates and proteins. If you take in more calories than you need you will get fat. Fibre, minerals, vitamins and water do not contain calories. They will not make you fat. But they will not give you energy either.

Carbohydrates

These are starchy or sugary foods. Examples are bread, oats, potato, pasta, rice, beans, root vegetables, sugar, glucose, sweets and candies. Some dieticians abbreviate carbohydrate to CHO. This can be confusing as Bill and Myra (whom I described in *Diabetes Beyond 40*) found out.

Bill and Myra were in their mid-seventies when Bill developed diabetes. They both listened carefully to the enthusiastic young dietician as she explained about Bill's diet. She wrote it all down for them and they took the diet sheet home to study carefully. They puzzled and puzzled over it. For every meal Bill was supposed to eat a strange food called CHO. Neither of them could remember what the dietician had said about CHO but it was obviously important. So Myra set out with her shopping bag to buy some. She tried two supermarkets and in each a helpful assistant searched along the shelves – no CHOs. She tried a delicatessen and two pharmacies. Finally a pharmacist explained that CHO was simply an abbreviation for carbohydrate!

Complex carbohydrates

These are also known as unrefined or starchy carbohydrates. The starch in bread, potato, pasta, rice, beans, oats and other similar foods is broken down by digestion into more simple carbohydrates such as glucose. As I explained in Chapter 5, these starchy carbohydrate foods are better for people with diabetes than sugary foods, because starches take a long time to be digested and release their glucose slowly.

Complex carbohydrates are often mixed with fibre in food. Fibre is the substance which stiffens plants and makes up their cell walls. It is not digested and remains in the bowel to act as roughage. There are two sorts of fibre – insoluble fibre and soluble fibre. Insoluble fibre is found in vegetables (e.g. cabbage, celery), bran, wholemeal bread, brown rice. It forms a tangle in which the starchy carbohydrate is embedded. Soluble fibre is that found in kidney beans, lentils, baked beans and other legumes. It forms a glue-like solution containing the starchy carbohydrate. Soluble fibre is especially good at improving glucose balance in people with diabetes.

Work in Oxford and elsewhere showed, in people with diabetes, that a diet in which 50–60 per cent of all calories are eaten as starchy high fibre carbohydrate produced better glucose control than the old

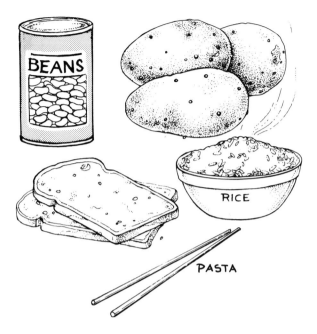

Complex carbohydrate foods

low carbohydrate diet. So most of what you eat should be starchy, high fibre carbohydrate.

Simple carbohydrates

These are also known as refined or sugary carbohydrates. The word 'sugar' is confusing. The granulated sugar we buy from the supermarket to put in our tea or cook with is sucrose, but the word sugar is also used more loosely in conversation to mean anything that tastes sweet. People talk about their blood sugar when they mean their blood glucose.

Simple carbohydrates include sucrose (which is made up of two glucoses), glucose itself, fructose or fruit sugar, and foods containing these – sweets, candies, sweet drinks such as pop, soda, cola drinks, fruit, jelly (jello in America) and jams (jellies).

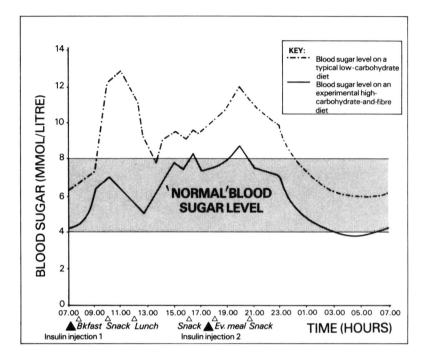

Improved diabetic control on a high carbohydrate fibre diet

Simple carbohydrates are digested and absorbed rapidly, producing a sudden peak of glucose in the bloodstream. However, if they are associated with large amounts of fibre (for example as part of a wholemeal bread and jam sandwich, or in an apple or pear) the glucose will be absorbed more slowly. For many years people with diabetes were told that they must never eat sucrose but they were allowed fruit freely. This was illogical as many fruits contain sucrose! Studies have shown that the blood glucose rises no more after meals containing small amounts of sucrose with large amounts of starchy, high-fibre carbohydrate than after a meal containing the same number of calories eaten as complex carbohydrates alone. If you want some sugar the British Diabetic Association suggest no more than 25 g a day (4 teaspoons of granulated sugar) eaten as part of a meal. In general, however, you should avoid eating sugar (granulated, icing, crystals, brown etc.) and foods containing it (cakes, candies, sweet biscuits etc.)

58

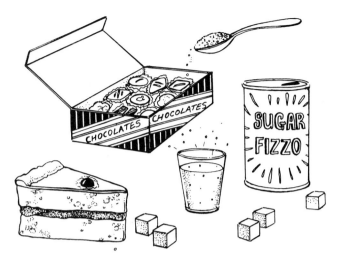

Foods containing simple sugars

Sweet fruits and honey contain fructose as well as sucrose. You can buy 'diabetic' foods in which the sucrose has been replaced by fructose. There is little evidence that long-term use of fructose is better than sucrose and it may, in fact, be worse. Fructose is broken down to compounds which may raise the blood glucose in people whose blood glucose is not optimally controlled. Furthermore, it may encourage a rise in one of the blood fats, triglyceride, which could be harmful long-term. The sensible course is to count fructose as a simple sugar like sucrose. Eat a moderate amount of natural fructose, as fruit for example, but do not eat extra fructose – there is no need to do so. You should eat lots of vegetables, both raw and cooked.

Avoid sugar in tea or coffee. Try to do without, or if you cannot, use an artificial sweetener in moderation – tiny quantities go a long way. Many people feel that aspartame tastes most like sugar. Use the smallest possible amount and try and do without if possible. Do not drink sweet drinks such as lemonade, colas, pop and other canned drinks. Use the 'Diet' versions in moderation. Try mineral waters or dilute real fruit juice with mineral water or carbonated water. Small amounts of undiluted fruit juice are all right.

Carbohydrate exchanges

In the past much emphasis was placed upon weighing food and calculating exchanges exactly. Such time-consuming precision is not necessary. However, at first, weighing and reading the contents may help you to learn about different foods. Some people find it helpful to know how much carbohydrate there is in different foods so that they can eat similar amounts at each meal time or snack time. The standard exchange is 10 grammes of glucose. Thus a medium-sized apple is considered to contain the equivalent carbohydrate of 10 grammes of glucose. However, the way in which the food is prepared (e.g. boiled potato, mashed potato, crisps, potato soup) and the state of your insides determines how rapidly each form of that particular food is digested and its carbohydrate content absorbed.

Research workers in Oxford, Canada and elsewhere have used a measure called glycaemic index to attempt to produce a more accurate comparison between carbohydrate foods. This compares the blood-glucose rise, under standard conditions, after a particular carbohydrate food, with a standard carbohydrate load. The glycaemic index of the same food may vary depending on how it is prepared. For example, the blood glucose will rise more after apple juice, than after cooked apple. It will rise least after eating a raw apple. This is why elaborate calculations of carbohydrate exchanges are misleading and unnecessary.

Proteins

These are found in meat such as chicken or lean beef, fish, milk, cheese, quorn, beans and pulses, soya, nuts and in cereal foods. They are rarely found on their own and often have fat with them. We need protein for growth and repair. It is especially important that children have enough protein to develop their muscles and grow up. About 10–20 per cent of dietary calories should come from protein.

In the old days, people with diabetes were encouraged to eat lots of protein because it did not make the blood glucose rise straightaway. (In times of insulin lack, however, the body breaks down its own protein stores to make glucose – this process is called gluconeogenesis.) Cheese, was 'free', in other words, they could eat as much as they wanted. Sadly, cheese is laden with fat and we now know that too much fat is bad for your heart and blood vessels (see page 148).

Eat some protein-containing foods each day. Vegetarians will get plenty of protein – it occurs in plants such as beans, peas and lentils as well as animals. Quorn is a useful meat substitute.

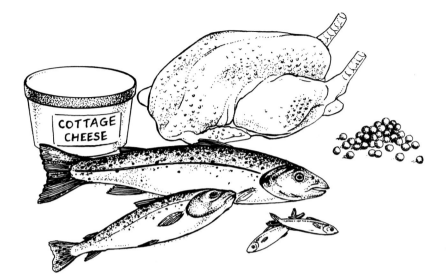

Protein foods

Fats

Fats are greasy or oily foods such as full cream milk, cream, butter, cheese, margarine, olive oil, sunflower oils, lard, dripping, meat fat. Nuts contain a lot of fat. There are also hidden fats in many foods – meat, cakes, biscuits, pastry, made-up meat dishes such as sausages and pork pies. Fats are very calorific – a small amount of fat gives you a lot of energy – or puts a lot of weight on.

People with diabetes need to be wary of fats for two reasons. Firstly, because many people with diabetes are trying to lose weight. Secondly, because people with diabetes often have high blood-fat concentrations. You should try to reduce your fat intake until less than 35 per cent of your daily calories comes from fat.

Buy low fat spreads rather than butter, use low fat yoghurt, eat lower fat cheeses (such as cottage cheese or Edam), and drink skimmed milk. Grill rather than fry, and drain the fat off oven-cooked meat. Reduce the amount of fat you use in cooking – do not add fat to stews or casseroles, and do not put it as a garnish on vegetables. Avoid rich puddings and gateaux. Scrape the spread onto your bread – any extra is wasted calories. Cut off visible fat on your meat. Do not have bread and butter and cheese – just have the bread and cheese.

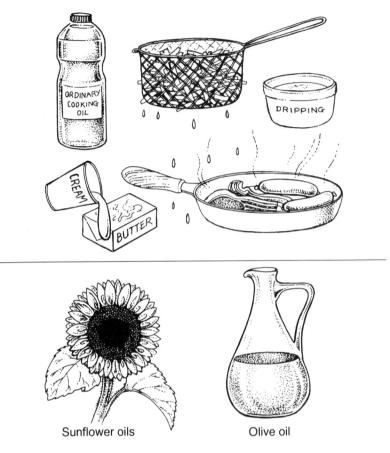

Sunflower oils   Olive oil

Saturated fats (above) polyunsaturated & monounsaturated (below)

Polyunsaturated and monounsaturated fats

Your most important aim is to reduce your total fat content. However, you should also look at the type of fats you are eating. Saturated fats, such as those found in butter, cream, cheese and the fat on meat, are particularly likely to fur up your arteries. Nuts also contain saturated fats. Polyunsaturated fats (such as sunflower spread) or monoun-saturated fats (such as olive oil) are better for you. You should also include oily fish as part of your diet.

Minerals and vitamins

If you eat a good mixture of the foods described above, you will not need to add vitamin or mineral pills to your diet.

One mineral of which we all tend to eat too much is salt or sodium chloride. There is no need to add extra salt at table. Many doctors believe that excessive salt intake elevates the blood pressure. It is sensible to restrict added salt to the minimum – there is plenty in our food.

There is one situation in which you may need extra salt and that is if you are dehydrated or salt and water deficient. Dehydration can be caused by excess sweating (e.g. by exercising very vigorously for a long time or in hot weather), diarrhoea or vomiting, or in severe insulin lack causing polyuria. In this situation it is better to drink slightly salty water or salt-replacement solutions such as Diorylate than plain water. Consommé or beef extract drinks are another source of salt in this situation. If the drink is unpalatable it is too salty.

Potassium is another mineral which we need in moderate amounts but which is harmful in excess. Most people do not need to worry about this – your body will keep you in perfect balance. However, if you are taking water pills (diuretics) for swollen ankles or shortness of breath, or as a treatment for high blood pressure, it is sensible to eat plenty of potassium-containing foods. These are citrus fruits, bananas, dried fruit such as apricots and tomatoes. Sometimes your doctor may give you potassium pills.

The majority of people obtain the vitamins they need from their food. If you are a very strict vegetarian or vegan you may become deficient in vitamin B_{12}. You will need to supplement this and there are now non-animal sources.

Drinks

If you add up the number of drinks of all kinds that you take in each day you may be surprised at the total. Most people drink a minimum of six glasses or cups of fluid a day. Doctors usually assume that an average-sized adult needs three litres of fluid a day. Someone who is eating and drinking normally will have some of this as separate drinks and the rest mixed in with the food – apples, soup, vegetables, for example. You can tell if you are taking in enough fluid by looking at your urine. It should be a pale straw colour. If it is very yellow or dark (what most of us would call concentrated) you need to drink more.

But which drink? You can have as much water as you want. Tea and coffee are fine in moderation, but too much will make you jittery because of the caffeine. Recent research suggests that there is no need to change to caffeine-free coffee to protect your heart, but some people like it as an alternative to ordinary coffee. Fruit juice is good in small amounts but watch the sugar content. Check the labels of canned drinks – some of them have added sucrose or glucose. Some people like beef extract drinks or vegetable juices – watch the salt content. Milk shakes and yoghurt drinks are often rather fatty and sugary.

Alcohol

Having diabetes does not stop you drinking alcohol, but stick to the commonsense limits. These are 14 units a week for women and 21 units a week for men. A unit of alcohol is a half-pint of beer or lager, a standard measure of spirit or a wine-glass full of wine. Be careful about low-sugar lagers. They have been brewed on to convert more of the sugar to alcohol. Low-alcohol lagers and wines may contain a lot of sugar. Choose a wine or lager which is low in both sugar and alcohol. Never drink on an empty stomach.

Monty had clinched a highly successful deal. He had a drink in the hotel bar with his boss before walking home. Because he has insulin-treated diabetes he had a pint of low-sugar lager. Half-an-hour later a policeman found him staggering across a road. Because Monty's breath smelled of alcohol the officer thought that he was drunk and took him to a police station. He became more and more confused and they put him in a cell to 'sober up'. Fortunately, the custody sergeant searched his pockets and found his diabetic card and some glucose tablets. When they had cured his hypoglycaemia they took him home.

Hypoglycaemia or a low blood glucose is described on pages 101 to 113. Alcohol prevents the liver from releasing glucose from its stores and can cause hypoglycaemia in non-diabetics.

There is now a wide range of non-alcoholic drinks. Many people space out alcoholic drinks with these. Check the label as some of these are quite sugary.

If you drink very heavily for a long time you can damage your pancreas so badly that it causes diabetes.

'Diabetic' foods and other special foods or additives

'Diabetic' foods There is no need to buy expensive 'diabetic' foods. Advertisements for such foods have now been banned from the British Diabetic Association's magazine. 'Diabetic' foods are made with fructose or sorbitol rather than glucose or sucrose. As discussed above, there is no evidence that fructose is better for diabetics than glucose and it contains the same number of calories so it cannot be used as part of a weight-reducing diet. Sorbitol is broken down to fructose. It causes bowel upsets if large amounts (i.e. more than 30 g) are eaten. If you desperately want some chocolate, have a little bit of ordinary chocolate after a mixed meal. Look on the packet for the carbohydrate content and remember to include the chocolate in your 25 g of sucrose for that day.

Artificial sweeteners These can make soft drinks and puddings more palatable. You need only tiny amounts. Aspartame is the most natural tasting sweetener and saccharine is rarely used nowadays. Use sweeteners sparingly. It is better to learn how to enjoy less sweet tastes.

'Health' foods, pills and additives I once met a man who was taking 40 different doses of 'health pills' a day. I had to tell him that he might well be overdosing on some compounds. Others were probably harmless but unnecessary.

Most of us get all we need to keep fit from a mixed diet. We do not need additives. If you are tempted to buy from a health food shop, check the labels carefully. A herbal remedy may not have undergone the stringent tests and manufacturing controls demanded of the pharmaceutical industry. One herbal remedy used in diabetes care was Goats Rue. The active component of this is metformin – now manufactured as a glucose-lowering drug (see page 76).

The diabetic diet has changed

Those of you who have had diabetes for many years, or who have had relatives with diabetes may have found this section confusing. Ideas about diabetic diets have changed considerably over the years. In the 18th century Rollo advocated a low calorie diet containing rancid meat! In the first part of the 20th century the only treatment for diabetes was starvation with severe carbohydrate restriction. This idea that diabetics could not eat carbohydrate persisted for some years after the discovery of insulin. Unless people were overweight they were allowed unlimited fats and proteins. Nowadays we know that too much fat is harmful and that people need lots of complex carbohydrate mixed with fibre for a healthy diet.

HOW MUCH YOU EAT

When you eat food it is either used as fuel straightaway, or stored for future use in one of the body's fuel depots. One of these is the liver – another is fat. So if you eat more than your body needs you get fat. To paraphrase Mr Micawber:

- Daily intake 2000 calories, daily expenditure 2000 calories, result happiness;
- Daily intake 2500 calories, daily expenditure 2000 calories, result obesity.

So, it should be simple to lose weight. Eat less than you need each day and you will lose weight. But we all know that it is not as easy as that. Food is nice. Food is friendly. It is comforting. It fills our tummies. Eating less can make you feel hungry. Feeling hungry is not nice. It can be very hard to cut down.

A further problem is that everyone is different in their fuel needs. We all know some really skinny person who eats like a horse and never puts weight on. We also know people (perhaps us) who have difficulty losing weight even if they eat very small helpings. So how does one lose weight?

The first step is to be honest with yourself. Write down every single thing you eat and drink for a week. And write down how much (e.g. how many spoonfuls of cereal or pudding, how many slices of bread). Sit down and look at that list.

1. Avoid unnecessary calories Are you eating anything that you don't actually like? If yes, then stop – why eat food you do not enjoy? Are you eating other people's leftovers – the children's for example? If yes, stop. You are not a garbage truck.

2. Avoid mechanical eating Do you sit in front of the television dipping into a bag of crisps? Or eat a packet of biscuits while you are typing? Are you actually enjoying each mouthful? If you must chew while you are doing things, try sugar-free chewing gum, or celery.

3. Regain control Is most of your eating out or in your home? If you are eating out, you often have less control over your food. Could you take a packed lunch rather than eat greasy canteen chips? Is there a fruit and vegetable shop you could choose rather than the burger bar? If you are eating in, can you control what you eat? Does someone else

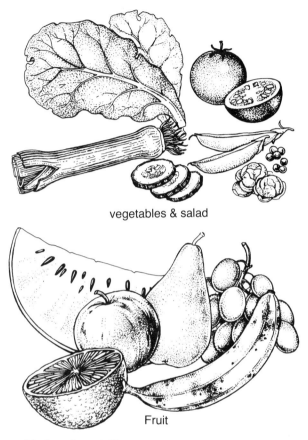

vegetables & salad

Fruit

Eat plenty of fruit and vegetables

cook for you? Involve them in your need to lose weight. All of us like to see someone enjoying our cooking, and there is a natural tendency to encourage second helpings. Explain that you are not rejecting them or their cooking, but following doctor's orders to lose weight. (In fact, one study showed that the wives of diabetic men are much more likely to change their own eating to help their husbands stick to their diet, than husbands of diabetic women.)

4. Say no This may be the hardest part. Start saying no. No to fatty foods. No to sugary foods. No to second helpings.

5. Say yes Go through your diet sheet with the dietician and focus on foods you like that you are allowed. Look at less fattening ways of cooking other favourite foods. Make sure that you have as many of the foods that you like as possible.

6. Eat less Have smaller portions. Use a smaller plate so that the helpings look bigger. Put a teaspoonful back each time.

7. Fill up on non-fattening vegetables – these include artichokes, asparagus, green beans, broccoli, Brussels sprouts, carrots, pumpkin, radish, spinach, swede, watercress, marrow, lettuce, cabbage, cucumber, celery, tomato, courgette, marrow, and onions.

8. Stay busy Occupy your mind so that you are not thinking of food all the time. Learn new hobbies. Try to avoid situations when you will feel pressure to over eat.

9. Exercise Burn off some of the fat. See chapter 17.

10. Be honest with yourself and your dietician or doctor. The only person you harm with untruths is yourself. I see overweight people who assure me they are sticking to their diet as they sit there with shopping bags of calorie-rich food at their feet! Many people swear that they are eating tiny amounts of food 'barely enough to keep a bird alive, doctor'. But studies have shown that people who say this and cannot lose weight are actually overeating – often nibbling continuously. You may not even realise you are doing it. So watch yourself.

Doreen is 32 and weighs 18 stone (252 pounds). She is on a diet. This is what Doreen thought she had eaten on Monday.

Breakfast half a grapefruit, black coffee, one slice toast with low fat spread and one teaspoon marmalade.

Lunch chicken sandwich (2 slices bread, low fat spread), tomato, lettuce, cucumber; apple.

Cup of tea.

Dinner weight watcher's frozen meal 240 calories. Perrier water. Lemon water ice (made with artificial sweetener). Coffee.

This is what Doreen actually ate:

Made mother's early morning tea – ate broken biscuit.

Got children's breakfast – ate piece of toast while making theirs.

Breakfast half a grapefruit, black coffee, one slice toast with low fat spread and one teaspoon marmalade (licked marmalade spoon).

Out shopping tasted cheeses at display in supermarket – five mouthfuls. Met friend and had cup of coffee with cream in department store.

Lunch chicken sandwich (2 slices bread, low fat spread), tomato, lettuce, cucumber; large spoonful of mayonnaise; apple.

Afternoon job in office Julie's birthday. Ate most of a slice of birthday cake. Cup of tea.

Prepared childrens' tea. Ate several peanuts and the sausage that burst in the frying pan.

Dinner weight watcher's frozen meal 240 calories. Perrier water. Drank half a glass of husband's wine. Lemon water ice (made with artificial sweetener). Coffee.

Grapes.

Midnight Very hungry. Went downstairs and ate two biscuits.

10. **Don't give up** If you have a set-back, just keep trying. Everyone is human. Remember, every ounce lost is a step towards becoming slimmer.

Diabetes treatment and weight loss

If you are overweight, weight loss is part of your diabetes treatment. However, it is important to adjust the dose of glucose-lowering pills or insulin if you start eating less and losing weight. If you do not reduce your insulin as your weight falls you are likely to become hypoglycaemic.

Metric

Height without shoes (m)	Men Weight without clothes (kg)			Women Weight without clothes (kg)		
	Acceptable average	Acceptable weight range	Obese	Acceptable average	Acceptable weight range	Obese
1.45				46.0	42–53	64
1.48				46.5	42–54	65
1.50				47.0	43–55	66
1.52				48.5	44–57	68
1.54				49.5	44–58	70
1.56				50.4	45–58	70
1.58	55.8	51–64	77	51.3	46–59	71
1.60	57.6	52–65	78	52.6	48–61	73
1.62	58.6	53–66	79	54.0	49–62	74
1.64	59.6	54–67	80	55.4	50–64	77
1.66	60.6	55–69	83	56.8	51–65	78
1.68	61.7	56–71	85	58.1	52–66	79
1.70	63.5	58–73	88	60.0	53–67	80
1.72	65.0	59–74	89	61.3	55–69	83
1.74	66.5	60–75	90	62.6	56–70	84
1.76	68.0	62–77	92	64.0	58–72	86
1.78	69.4	64–79	95	65.3	59–74	89
1.80	71.0	65–80	96			
1.82	72.6	66–82	98			
1.84	74.2	67–84	101			
1.86	75.8	69–86	103			
1.88	77.6	71–88	106			
1.90	79.3	73–90	108			
1.92	81.0	75–93	112			

Non-metric

Height without shoes (ft,in)	Men Weight without clothes (lb)			Women Weight without clothes (lb)		
	Acceptable average	Acceptable weight range	Obese	Acceptable average	Acceptable weight range	Obese
4 10				102	92–119	143
4 11				104	94–122	146
5 0				107	96–125	150
5 1				110	99–128	154
5 2	123	112–141	169	113	102–131	152
5 3	127	115–144	173	116	195–134	161
5 4	130	118–148	178	120	108–138	166
5 5	133	121–152	182	123	111–142	170
5 6	136	124–156	187	128	114–146	175
5 7	140	128–161	193	132	118–150	180
5 8	145	132–166	199	136	122–154	185
5 9	149	136–170	204	140	126–158	190
5 10	153	140–174	209	144	130–163	196
5 11	158	144–179	215	148	134–168	202
6 0	162	148–184	221	152	138–173	208
6 1	166	152–189	227			
6 2	171	156–194	233			
6 3	176	160–199	239			
6 4	181	164–204	245			

Guidelines for body weight

70

Careful blood glucose monitoring can help you here. A benefit of weight loss is often lower doses of glucose-lowering treatment.

ASIAN FOODS

If you enjoy sharing traditional food with family and friends in the community, or have to obey religious rules about food and drink, you can still eat a diet that suits your diabetes. Much of what has been said already in this chapter applies. Traditional Asian diets usually contain healthy amounts of vegetables, fruit, and carbohydrate such as rice (use brown rice), pulses such as lentils (e.g. dal), beans (e.g. rajam) and chickpeas (e.g. cholas, cabuli chanas), breads (chapatti – use wholemeal flour). Avoid sweet foods such as jelabi, kulfi and gur. Some dishes (e.g. halva) could be sweetened with aspartame or saccharine. Pay attention to the cooking of your food. It is important not to use too much fat such as ghee or the various cooking oils. What oil you do use should be carefully measured and high in polyunsaturated fats (e.g. sunflower oil) or monounsaturated fats (e.g. olive oil). Some meat dishes and vegetable preparations (e.g. aubergines) are cooked in fat, and it is often used to prepare some carbohydrate foods, such as nan, poppadums, poorata and pooris. Some dishes such as samosas are fried. Consider different ways of cooking such as stir-fry cooking using very little oil. Milk, yoghurt and butter (ghee) are full of saturated fat, so use skimmed milk, very low fat yoghurt, and avoid butter. When making tea do not boil the milk and sugar with it but use sweeteners such as canderal after heating if you need a sweet flavour. Avoid yoghurt drinks such as lassi (unless made with low fat yoghurt). Nuts contain a lot of fat too. You can eat whatever spices you wish. Be careful with herbal remedies or foods, they may contain medicines which interact with your treatment from the hospital. Karela lowers the blood glucose, so tell your doctor if you are eating this vegetable or any herbal preparation.

Fasting

Many religions have fast days or periods of restrained eating. Ramadan or other fasting periods can be observed safely if you wish although your religious guide may grant you exemption on the grounds of ill health. Discuss this with your diabetes adviser before you begin your fast. You may need to reduce your pills or insulin, or to take them only during the hours of darkness when food is permitted,

71

for example. Failure to work out exactly what to do about your treatment may cause hypoglycaemia (see page 101) during periods of fasting.

SUMMARY

- A diet is what you eat.
- Your body cannot cope with sugary foods whose carbohydrate is quickly absorbed.
- Eat plenty of starchy, fibrous carbohydrate which is digested slowly. Your body can cope with that.
- Eat as little fat as possible.
- Eat a small amount of protein.
- Avoid manufactured 'diabetic' foods.
- Drink alcohol in moderation.
- Do not eat excess salt.
- Eat less of everything if you are overweight.
- Enjoy what you eat.

8

GLUCOSE-LOWERING PILLS

If dietary measures do not return your blood glucose to normal your doctor will probably prescribe glucose-lowering pills (also called oral hypoglycaemic agents). The indications for insulin treatment are listed in Chapter 9. Glucose-lowering pills will only work if your pancreas is still making some insulin. They will not help you if you do not keep to your diabetic diet.

There are two kinds of glucose-lowering pill – sulphonylureas, which were developed in the late 1950s, and metformin.

SULPHONYLUREAS

Currently used sulphonylureas

Chlorpropamide was the first. It is still used although gradually being replaced by newer sulphonylureas. It is extremely long-acting – over 24 hours – so should be taken once a day at the same time each day.

Glibenclamide is the most commonly used sulphonylurea. It is still quite long-acting but is taken in split doses at meal times. Glibenclamide enters the islet cells themselves and stays there for many hours.

Tolbutamide is a shorter-acting first generation drug. The tablets are quite large.

More recent sulphonylureas include gliclazide which is being used increasingly. Its effect is similar in duration to glibenclamide but it produces a more 'normal' insulin response to glucose than glibenclamide. It also reduces blood stickiness which may reduce blood vessel complications of diabetes.

Glucose-lowering pills

Name of pill (Drug co. names in brackets)	Dosage range (per 24 hours)	Duration of action (Approximate)
chlorpropamide (Diabenese)	50–500 mg	36 hours or longer
glibenclamide (Daonil, Semi-daonil, Euglucon)	2.5–15 mg	5–20 hours
gliclazide (Diamicron)	40–320 mg	5–20 hours
glipizide (Glibenese, Minodiab)	2.5–40 mg	4–12 hours
gliquidone (Glurenorm)	15–160 mg	4–5 hours
metformin (Glucophage, Orabet)	500–2000 mg	?8–12 hours
tolazamide (Tolanase)	100–750 mg	7–24 hours
tolbutamide	500–2000 mg	3–8 hours

This is a general guide. It should be noted that some doctors use larger doses of some drugs and that the duration of action may vary.

Others include glipizide (short-acting) which some doctors use instead of tolbutamide. Glibornuride, gliquidone and glymidine are less often used. Other sulphonylureas are being developed.

How do they work?

The sulphonylureas work in several ways. They boost insulin release by the pancreas in response to a glucose load. They also have effects in the liver and tissues, helping the insulin to work more effectively at receptor level and perhaps in the cells (page 34).

When not to use sulphonylureas

Not at all for insulin-requiring diabetes, in pregnancy, for breast-feeding mothers.

With caution in liver disease, kidney disease, adrenal insufficiency, thyroid disease.

Drugs which interfere with sulphonylureas or vice versa

There are many including sulphonamide antibiotics (e.g. Septrin) and chloramphenicol, phenylbutazone, ibuprofen and similar drugs, aspirin, probenecid, warfarin, beta blockers, monoamine oxidase inhibitors, sulphinpyrazone, barbiturates. Thiazides and steroids may increase the blood glucose.

Side-effects

The most obvious side-effect is hypoglycaemia. Others include allergic reactions like skin rashes, and gastrointestinal upsets – nausea or bowel symptoms, for example. Alcohol causes flushing with some, especially chlorpropamide. Rarely, they cause liver damage or abnormalities of blood cells. In most instances the side-effects disappear once the drug is stopped. In the early 1960s the American University Group Diabetes Program suggested that tolbutamide use was associated with an increased risk of heart disease. However, this study has since been criticised and most doctors in Britain and America continue to recommend sulphonylureas. They rarely upset people and are taken by millions world-wide.

Hypoglycaemia on sulphonylureas

Obviously these pills are meant to lower your blood glucose. However, if you take more pills than you need, eat too little or exercise unexpectedly your glucose may fall lower than you want. You may become hypoglycaemic. The symptoms and signs of hypoglycaemia are detailed in Chapter 10. If you suspect you are hypoglycaemic you must test your blood glucose, or if this is at all difficult or you feel very unwell, eat some glucose immediately. It is extremely important to follow this up with a good meal. Then contact your diabetes adviser. Because you still have the sulphonylurea in your bloodstream, it will encourage your pancreas to keep releasing insulin every time your blood glucose rises. So you may keep becoming hypoglycaemic. With chlorpropamide severely hypoglycaemic people can have recurrent glucose falls for a day or more, until the drug has worn off.

Glibenclamide is the commonest cause of hypoglycaemia in pill-treated people – probably because it is prescribed often and can last for 20 hours. One in three people taking glibenclamide report hypoglycaemic episodes so you must be alert for this. Several companies make glibenclamide and there may be differences in availability of the drug in the body from different preparations. The

75

high frequency of hypoglycaemia on glibenclamide is why some doctors prefer gliclazide nowadays.

METFORMIN

This is the only drug of its class still in use. It is prescribed in a dose of 500–1700 mg daily in divided doses (some doctors give up to 3000 mg although rarely in Britain). It does not boost pancreatic insulin production and so is unlikely to cause hypoglycaemia unless taken in overdose. It helps insulin to work in the tissues and reduces glucose absorption from the bowel.

Metformin is particularly useful in overweight people as it helps them to lose weight (if they stick to their weight-reducing diet). It can cause a loss of appetite as well as reducing glucose absorption.

When not to use metformin

Not at all in pregnancy, breast feeding; people who drink too much alcohol; those with severe disease of kidneys, liver, heart or lungs

With caution in elderly people

Drugs which interfere with metformin and vice versa

Warfarin.

Side-effects

These are more common than with sulphonylureas but can usually be avoided by starting treatment with very small doses so that the body gets used to the metformin. Side-effects may include lack of appetite, nausea, vomiting and diarrhoea, an odd taste in the mouth, wind, indigestion. Rarely anaemia due to vitamin B_{12} or folate malabsorption may occur. The most dangerous side effect is lactic acidosis – a severe acid derangement of blood chemistry. This is very uncommon and usually occurs in people who have kidney failure, a very low blood pressure or who have very severe infections – in other words, those who are very ill.

COMBINATION TREATMENT

If your blood glucose cannot be controlled with one of these agents alone, combining it with another may be successful because they work in different ways. In Britain many people take glibenclamide (nowadays often gliclazide) and metformin.

PROBLEMS WITH PILLS

Failure to control the blood glucose

If combination treatment and a careful diabetic diet do not maintain good blood glucose balance you need insulin. Although no-one likes injecting themselves with insulin it is much better not to delay starting treatment – you will feel very much better within days and it is not as awful as you imagine (see Chapter 9).

Vomiting and other illness

If you cannot keep your tablets down or have diarrhoea (which may mean that you do not absorb them), call your doctor. In the meantime check your blood glucose at least 6-hourly, and preferably more often. If you are too ill to measure your own glucose you need to be in hospital. Infections and other illness push the blood glucose up – you may need insulin to help to control it at this time. Vomiting is a danger signal in diabetes – it may reflect an illness that causes your blood glucose to rise, it may stop you having your treatment or it may be due to a high glucose and major chemical imbalance. Call for help early.

Failure to control the blood glucose

You may simply need more pills (assuming you are sticking to your diabetic diet). Ask your doctor or diabetes adviser for guidelines so that you can increase you pills (within the safe dosage range) if your blood glucose levels rise.

You may be on the maximum dose of pills. The blood glucose may rise temporarily because of an illness or operation. A few days or weeks of insulin treatment will solve this. However, as the years go by, the pancreas produces less and less insulin until finally the pills can work no longer. When this happens, no amount of adjustment of the type of pills or their dose will help and you need insulin injections. This is not a major problem. If you wait, 'just one more try with the pills', 'I'll try really hard with the diet', you may find yourself suffering all the symptoms of untreated diabetes, feeling ill. If you need insulin have it so that you will start feeling better quickly.

What should you know about your pills?

1. Their name: the proper name (e.g. glibenclamide) and any trade name (e.g. Daonil).

2. What they are for: lowering the blood glucose.

3. When to take them: before or with the meal for sulphonylureas and with or after the meal for metformin. Make sure you know the correct mealtimes.

4. How much to take: be careful – some are marketed in different strengths. So you need to know the size of your pills and your dose in milligrammes (mgs) or grammes (gs). (One g = 1000 mg) 40 mg gliclazide is half an 80 mg pill; 160 mg gliclazide is two 80 mg pills. You may need to take a different dose morning and evening. (You may be offended that I am spelling this out but mistakes often occur.)

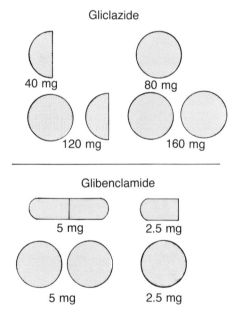

What are you taking? How much?

78

5. What unwanted effects may occur: hypoglycaemia with sulphonylureas; see pages 75 and 76 for other effects.

6. Possible interactions with other pills

7. How long to take them for: indefinitely unless you are told otherwise. This means making sure you get some more before your current supply runs out. Show the doctor the original bottle. Compare the pills the pharmacist gives you with the ones in your original bottle – they should be the same.

8. Cost: Diabetics on glucose-lowering pills are exempt from prescription charges in Britain.

9. Is your diabetic card correct? Carry it always.

10. If you are taking a sulphonylurea carry glucose with you always.

SUMMARY

- Glucose-lowering pills only work if you are still making some insulin of your own.
- Sulphonylureas lower the blood glucose effectively. They can cause hypoglycaemia.
- Metformin also lowers the blood glucose effectively. It may help overweight people lose weight.
- Make sure you know what you are taking, when, how much and what for.
- Carry a diabetic card.
- Carry glucose if taking sulphonylureas.
- Monitor your blood glucose concentration.
- Seek help early with vomiting illness, or other illness in which your blood glucose is rising.

9

INSULIN TREATMENT

If your body can no longer make sufficient insulin to keep your blood glucose normal, you need insulin treatment. Many people are frightened about this, but nowadays, you need not be worried. The injection itself hurts no more than a gnat bite and even small children can learn how to draw up and inject insulin. Furthermore, if you have a modern insulin pen, you do not even have to use a needle and syringe – just select the dose on your pen and slip the fine needle into a fold of skin and fat.

WHO NEEDS INSULIN?

People who have IDDM need insulin. This includes the majority of people whose diabetes comes on before the age of 30 years. If you make no insulin then no other treatment will work.

People who have failed to control their blood glucose with diet and glucose-lowering pills also need insulin. This treatment has failed because you are no longer making enough insulin for the pills to work. Note that I have said that the *treatment* has failed – not you. It is not your fault that your pancreas is failing to produce enough insulin. You will feel much better on insulin treatment, so do not put it off.

If your diabetes is usually controlled by diet alone or by diet and pills you may need insulin treatment temporarily when you are ill. Examples are during infections or operations or after accidents. In most cases you can return to your usual treatment once you have recovered.

Pregnant women who have diabetes which they cannot control by diet alone, or who usually take glucose-lowering tablets, must have insulin treatment until the baby has been born.

WHAT YOU NEED TO KNOW ABOUT INSULIN TREATMENT

Essential information

Write this down and carry it with you at all times. It is essential to your survival.

- The name of the insulin(s) your doctor has prescribed;
- The dose(s);
- When to inject it;
- Where to inject it;
- How to keep your insulin in good condition;
- Where to get your insulin from;
- The name of your insulin-injection system (i.e. which syringe and needle, or which pen);
- How to look after your insulin-injection system;
- Where to get your insulin-injection system from;
- How to use your insulin and your injection system;
- What to do if you feel odd or ill;
- Who to contact if you need help (day or night).

Desirable information

The essential information is minimal. It will not allow you to adjust your treatment yourself. Nor will it allow you to sort out many emergencies yourself. Further information will help you to understand how your treatment works and may well save you inconvenience or illness. As Dr Lawrence said, 'it is not enough that your doctor should put you on the proper lines of treatment. You must learn to follow it and carry it out yourself in your own home'. Learning as much as you can about your insulin and the way in which you use it and your body responds will make the difference between having to adapt your life to your treatment and adapting your treatment to suit your life. Information that it is desirable for you to have, therefore, covers the following:

- What type of insulin?
- How does it work?
- What effects does it have on the body?
- How can you adjust the dose and timing?
- What to do in emergencies?
- What other insulins and injection systems are there?

Because I believe that all of you will want to control your treatment, rather than have it control you, I will combine the essential and desirable information in the following sections.

INSULIN

Types of insulin

Clear The insulin that your body used to make was a clear colourless substance. This type of insulin is produced as a clear water-like liquid. It used to be called soluble insulin (regular insulin in America). Hypurin soluble is one example. Nowadays most clear insulins are called neutral. Some trade names are Actrapid, Humulin S (Humulin R in America), and Velosulin. You can always recognise a soluble insulin because it is a completely clear solution. This sort of insulin works fast. It is the only one which can be injected directly into the bloodstream (this is only done in hospital). There it starts to work within minutes. Injected under the skin it starts to work within half an hour and most have their greatest effect between two and six hours. Some, like Humulin S, have an earlier maximal effect. Research is progressing with ultrafast insulins but these are not yet available for general use.

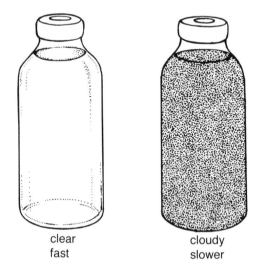

clear
fast

cloudy
slower

Insulin

Clear insulins will deal with one meal eaten within 15–30 minutes of injection. Some people may have an injection of clear insulin before each meal.

Cloudy These insulins have all been treated to delay their onset of action after injection. So, just by looking at the bottle or cartridge of insulin, you can tell whether it is fast-acting (clear) or slower-acting (cloudy). Some of these insulins are slowed down by using crystalline forms, others by adding protamine and others by incorporating zinc. One of the problems with the cloudy insulins is that their duration of action may vary from person to person. An insulin that lasts 24 hours in one person may need to be given twice daily in someone else. In general the following insulins are usually medium-acting and are therefore given twice a day: Humulin I, Isophane, Insulatard, Protaphane, Semitard. Monotard comes somewhere in between. These insulins are usually considered longer-acting and are often given once daily: Lentard, Lente, Humulin Zn. These insulins are usually considered very long-acting and are only given once daily: Hypurin Protamine Zinc and Ultratard.

Fixed-proportion mixtures These are mixtures of clear and isophane insulins provided by the manufacturer. They include Actraphane, Humulin M1, Humulin M2, Humulin M3, Humulin M4, Initard, Mixtard and Rapitard. If you increase the dose of one of these insulins the dose of both the short and medium-acting components will increase.

How is insulin made? Human, pig and beef insulin

Originally the only source of insulin was animal pancreas – either beef or pig. The need for good supplies of pig pancreas meant that much insulin was made in Denmark. Beef insulin is rarely used today. It is less like human insulin than the porcine variety which differs in only one tiny detail.

About ten years ago, insulin became the first drug to be manufactured using genetic engineering. Harmless bacteria were made to produce human insulin by altering their genetic material. The bacteria were then killed and the insulin purified. This meant that people with diabetes were no longer dependent upon animals for their insulin supply. It also meant that they could, at last, have the insulin that their bodies would have been making were they not diabetic. Because animal insulins are 'foreign' to the body, antibodies (page 33) are

Preparation		Manufacturer	Strength i.u./ml 100	Species	Onset, peak activity and duration of action in hours (approx)
Neutral Insulin Injection	Neutral	Evans	●	🐄	
	Human Actrapid (pyr)	Novo Nordisk	●	🧍	
	Human Velosulin (emp)	Novo Nordisk Wellcome	●	🧍	
	Humulin S (prb)	Lilly	●	🧍	
	Hypurin Neutral	CP Pharm	●	🐄	
	Pur-In Neutral (emp)	Fisons Hosp. Prod.	●	🧍	
	Velosulin	Novo Nordisk Wellcome	●	🐖	
Biphasic Insulin Injection*	Human Actraphane (pyr)	Novo Nordisk	●	🧍	
	Human Initard 50/50 (emp)	Novo Nordisk Wellcome	●	🧍	
	Human Mixtard 30/70 (emp)	Novo Nordisk Wellcome	●	🧍	
	Humulin M1 (prb)	Lilly	●	🧍	
	Humulin M2 (prb)	Lilly	●	🧍	
	Humulin M3 (prb)	Lilly	●	🧍	
	Humulin M4 (prb)	Lilly	●	🧍	
	Initard 50/50	Novo Nordisk Wellcome	●	🐖	
	Mixtard 30/70	Novo Nordisk Wellcome	●	🐖	
	Penmix 10/90 (pyr)	Novo Nordisk	●	🧍	
	Penmix 20/80 (pyr)	Novo Nordisk	●	🧍	
	Penmix 30/70 (pyr)	Novo Nordisk	●	🧍	
	Penmix 40/60 (pyr)	Novo Nordisk	●	🧍	
	Penmix 50/50 (pyr)	Novo Nordisk	●	🧍	
	Pur-In Mix 50/50 (emp)	Fisons Hosp. Prod.	●	🧍	
	Pur-In Mix 25/75 (emp)	Fisons Hosp. Prod.	●	🧍	
	Pur-In Mix 15/85 (emp)	Fisons Hosp. Prod.	●	🧍	
	Rapitard MC	Novo Nordisk	●	🐖+🐄 25% 75%	
Insulin Zinc Suspension (Amorphous)	Semitard MC	Novo Nordisk	●	🐖	
Isophane Insulin Injection	Isophane (NPH)	Evans	●	🐄	
	Human Insulatard (emp)	Novo Nordisk Wellcome	●	🧍	
	Human Protaphane (pyr)	Novo Nordisk	●	🧍	
	Humulin I (prb)	Lilly	●	🧍	
	Hypurin Isophane	CP Pharm	●	🐄	
	Insulatard	Novo Nordisk Wellcome	●	🐖	
	Pur-In Isophane (emp)	Fisons Hosp. Prod.	●	🧍	
Insulin Zinc Suspension (Mixed)	Lente	Evans	●	🐄	
	Human Monotard (pyr)	Novo Nordisk	●	🧍	
	Humulin Lente (prb)	Lilly	●	🧍	
	Hypurin Lente	CP Pharm	●	🐄	
	Lentard MC	Novo Nordisk	●	🐖+🐄 30% 70%	
Insulin Zinc Suspension (Crystalline)	Human Ultratard (pyr)	Novo Nordisk	●	🧍	
	Humulin Zn (prb)	Lilly	●	🧍	
Protamine Zinc Insulin Injection	Hypurin Protamine Zinc	CP Pharm	●	🐄	

Scale: 0 2 4 6 8 10 12 14 16 18 20 22 24 26 28 30 32 34

(prb)-produced from proinsulin synthesised by bacteria using recombinant DNA technology
(pyr)-produced from a precursor synthesised by yeast using recombinant DNA technology
(emp)-produced by enzymatic modification of porcine insulin
*Speed of onset is proportional to amount of soluble insulin

Duration of action of different insulins

84

produced to the insulin which may necessitate increasingly larger doses of insulin to achieve the same glucose-lowering effect. Antibody formation may also cause variability in response to insulin. It has been suggested that these antibodies may be implicated in tissue damage. High antibody levels have been linked with the formation of big dents at injection sites (see page 95). (Antibodies can be made to human insulin too but much less often.) Modern highly purified insulins (from whatever origin) are less likely to cause antibody formation than older insulins. Genetically engineered insulin made by bacteria is denoted by 'crb' or 'prb' on the label. Yeasts can be used – 'pyr' on the label. It has also proved possible to modify porcine insulin using enzymes – 'emp' on the label. About 80 per cent of insulin-dependent diabetics in Britain now use human insulin and use of animal insulins is declining.

Strength All insulin in Britain is provided in a concentration of 100 units per millilitre. It is called U100 insulin. Other countries may have different strengths so beware if you try to obtain insulin abroad. You must use U100 syringes to give U100 insulin.

Preservative All insulin contains preservative to keep it sterile until the expiry date. This is why it smells slightly antiseptic and why you can keep sticking your needle into the bottle without infecting the insulin.

How is insulin packaged

Insulin usually comes in bottles with a self-sealing rubber bung. Every bottle is labelled with the name, and expiry date, among other information. Every time you obtain a new bottle of insulin and every time you use it, check that it is the right sort of insulin for you (if you are taking Humulin S and Humulin I, make sure you have not been given Humulin M1 or Humulin M2, for example), and check that it has not expired.

Increasingly, insulin is provided in cartridges. These are about the same size as ink cartridges and have a self-sealing rubber bung at one end (which will be penetrated by the double-ended pen-needle) and the plug which will be depressed by the pen plunger at the other end. It is possible to get insulin out of a cartridge using an ordinary syringe and needle but this should only be done in an emergency (e.g. broken pen and no back-up insulin) and is not to be recommended. As with insulin bottles make sure that you have the correct insulin and it is within its expiry date.

Because insulin is a protein it is digested if swallowed. However researchers are trying to put insulin into capsules which release their insulin only in the large bowel, beyond the reach of digestive enzymes. However, there are still many problems to be overcome, including that of ensuring good absorption and accurate dosage. These problems also arise with intranasal insulin – insulin which is sniffed up the nose. Both these ways of administering insulin are experimental and seem unlikely to replace insulin injections. Insulin-producing islet cells can also be implanted into the liver and other tissues – this means that they can produce insulin in the body. Several people with diabetes have received islet cell transplants but this remains a research technique. It is difficult to obtain enough pure islets and they have to be protected from rejection by your body. So for the time being, if you need insulin, it must be by injection.

How to look after your insulin

Insulin is a protein. This means that, like an egg, it is permanently altered by freezing or heating. But while you can still eat a previously frozen or cooked egg, insulin which has been altered in this way is useless.

Some researchers were testing a new type of insulin. A large batch was produced abroad and flown in specially. The cargo handlers unloaded the plane and left the containers on the tarmac to be collected later. It snowed and all the insulin froze. The entire consignment was worthless.

Bill is a sales representative and travels a lot. One day he nearly forgot his insulin. His wife ran after him and handed the bottles through the car window. He put them on the dashboard. He left the car parked in the sun all day. It was one of the hottest days of the year. The business trip lasted several days and although Bill stuck to his diet and his usual doses of insulin, his blood glucose went up and up and he started to feel thirsty. It was not until he returned home and started a fresh supply of insulin that he began to feel better. Eventually he realised that the insulin he took on his trip must have been damaged by heating in the sun.

Your can carry your current bottle(s) around with you and most insulin-pen users will carry their pen in their pocket. The insulin will not go off. However you must protect your insulin from freezing or cooking when you travel. Keep all your spare insulin in the fridge between 2° and 10°C. It is usually safest to keep it well away from the freezing compartment. Always, always have at least one spare bottle or cartridge in your house, or baggage if travelling. If you use a pen you should also have a bottle of insulin and a syringe and needle just in case of pen loss, damage or malfunction. Remember that if your bag is stolen you could lose your insulin. Consider keeping it in a safe pocket when travelling.

Although your insulin is self-sterilising it is sensible to keep it clean. This means cleaning the bung before inserting the needle. Some people use alcohol-impregnated swabs but there are sprays or bottles of alcohol or other antiseptics. Ask your doctor or nurse which they advise.

INSULIN-INJECTION SYSTEMS

Syringes

When I first became interested in diabetes, most insulin-treated patients were using glass syringes, many with re-usable needles. It was hard to keep the syringe clean, it was breakable and injections could be painful. Disposable syringes and fine disposable needles were used in hospital but were not available on outside prescription. Many clinics gave them out to patients when they could. Then, primarily as a result of efforts by the British Diabetic Association, supported by many individual patients and other concerned people, disposable syringes and needles became available on prescription. No-one needs to use a glass syringe nowadays.

The syringes are made by several companies. They are marketed with fixed or detachable needles. Those with a fixed needle are probably the most practical for the majority of patients. People who are injecting insulins which should not be mixed should have a separate needle and syringe. That way they can draw up each insulin separately and inject them through the same needle left in the skin. Few people will be giving insulin like this.

Syringes are very small (0.5 ml or 50 units) or small (1 ml or 100 units) and are marked in units of insulin. They are designed for single use only. Keep the syringe packet intact and dry until you use it or it will not be sterile.

It is your responsibility to keep your syringes and needles secure and to inform the police should they be lost or stolen. Similarly be careful about disposal. Your GP can prescribe needle clippers which will hold about a thousand needle ends and can then be thrown away safely. You can also obtain sharps boxes from the surgery or hospital depending on the system locally. Never throw a syringe and needle away in your domestic rubbish without first ensuring that no-one else could possibly prick themselves or (a sad reflection on our society) use it.

Insulin pens

Several insulin pens are available including Accupen, B-D Lilly pen, Novopen II, Penmix, Pur-in pen. They use an insulin cartridge with a self-sealing bung at one end and a rubber plug at the other. The disposable needle is double-ended – one end goes into the bung and the other, finer, needle goes into you. The insulin dose can be selected simply by depressing the plunger the right number of times (usually one press equals two units of insulin but check on your own pen), or by dialling up the correct dose and twisting or depressing the cap to inject the insulin. Your pen is easy to carry and easy to use and more and more people with diabetes have replaced their syringe and needle with one of these devices.

As there are several on the market and more on the way it is important to chose a pen which suits your needs. Some older pens are simply covers for a syringe with a replacement plunger. There are easier pens to use but this is the only system in which you can use any insulin. Otherwise, pens and insulins are not interchangeable. Each company makes a pen which uses only its own insulin. This is because the instruments have been designed and tested with specific insulins. So, unless you are prepared to change your insulin, you may find that

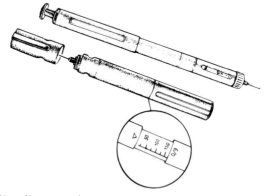

Two types of insulin pen syringes

the decision has been made for you. However, if you do have a choice, insist on actually handling several pens. Does it fit your hand? Can you dial up a dose and expel the insulin easily? Does the pen show you how much insulin you have used and how much is left? Can you correct mistakes before injection? Does the pen have a locking device so that insulin is not expressed until you wish it? Also find out what the back-up is like. What happens if you have a problem with the pen? Will the company give you another straightaway? Ideally you should have two pens – one for use and one spare but this may not be possible while pen numbers are limited.

Other devices

Several cannulae are available which can be left under the skin for a day or more. The insulin is injected into a self-sealing port. Most people find that injections are so trouble-free anyway that an indwelling device which could catch on clothes or become infected is not necessary. A few find it preferable.

There is also a syringe-based device which is continuously connected to such a cannula with tubing. The plunger can then be depressed the required amount at each meal to inject insulin.

Insulin jets use technology developed for mass immunisation to drive insulin through the skin under high pressure. This does not require an injection as such. Some people find these devices very helpful but others find that they get bruising at jet sites and that insulin oozes out again. They are more popular in America than in Britain.

Other aids include magnifiers to place over the markings on the syringe to aid vision when drawing up and guides to hide the needle. The advent of insulin pens has made insulin injections much easier and fewer people seem to have the problems with insulin administration which necessitated concealing devices.

Insulin pumps

Normally the pancreas releases insulin all the time – in tiny bursts every few seconds. Larger amounts are released when the blood glucouse rises. Thus it is simplistic to believe that even four injections of insulin a day can accurately mimic normal pancreatic function.

This led to the development of continuous subcutaneous insulin infusion (CSII) by pumps which are worn all the time. Pumps were very popular several years ago but have now become less so although many people still have them and value them. Some of the reasons for their decline in popularity are the need for very intensive supervision, the high frequency of problems (including ketoacidosis and, less commonly, severe hypoglycaemia), the discomfort, inconvenience and embarrassment of a box attached to a tube attached to a needle *in situ* for 24 hours a day, every day, and the demonstration that they provide no better glucose balance than very carefully monitored conventional insulin therapy. CSII is still an option for some patients who, despite frequent monitoring and appropriate insulin treatment and adjustment, cannot maintain good glucose balance. However, it is not an easy option and should be chosen carefully after thorough discussion with your diabetes adviser.

There are other, implantable, insulin pumps, for example intra-peritoneal (implanted into the abdominal cavity). Despite media excitement these are still at the experimental stage and are used only as a last resort. There are rare patients whose life has been saved by one of these devices but there are probably only a few such people in Britain with diabetes so severe as to need this drastic measure.

INSULIN TREATMENT PATTERNS

There are as many versions of insulin treatment as there are dia-betologists (doctors specialising in diabetes). Some patterns are more common than others. In general, once daily insulin is not an effective way of achieving good glucose balance and is reserved for elderly patients who have problems managing their condition or for very small children. Occasionally once daily insulin is used in people who have some residual pancreatic insulin production but not quite enough to keep their blood glucose normal. Many people use twice daily insulin and increasingly people are using pens before each meal.

In general, you need insulin for two types of glucose balance – coping with meals and helping with body housekeeping (dealing with the glucose produced by the body itself). Fast-acting, clear insulin copes with meals. Cloudy, longer-acting insulin copes with body housekeeping. Most people need about two thirds of their total daily insulin in the morning and one third in the early evening. About a third of your insulin will probably be fast-acting and about two thirds longer-acting. The type of insulin pattern you need must be tailored for you personally and no-one else. There is no right or wrong insulin pattern. Your final insulin pattern may be completely different from anything described in this book – if it gives you good glucose balance and you can manage it then that is the right insulin pattern for you.

Twice daily insulin

This is usually a combination of clear, fast-acting insulin mixed with cloudy medium-acting insulin given before breakfast and before the evening meal:

- Morning clear works until lunchtime;
- Morning cloudy works from lunch to evening meal;
- Evening clear works until bedtime;
- Evening cloudy works overnight until next morning.

Multiple pen injections with background insulin

This uses a cloudy, very long-acting insulin, (usually Ultratard) taken before bed as background to several pen injections of fast-acting clear insulin taken before each meal, whenever it is eaten:

- Pre-breakfast clear works until lunchtime;
- Pre-lunch clear works until evening meal;
- Pre-evening meal clear works until bedtime;
- Bedtime cloudy works overnight and into the next day.

Insulin should be injected about 20 minutes before eating but some people find that the genetically engineered clear insulins can be injected while sitting at the table as they start to act very quickly. You need to find your own best injection time.

DRAWING UP INSULIN

This is shown in the illustrations. Obviously, if you do not draw up the correct dose your insulin will not have the desired effect on your blood glucose. Insulin is very concentrated and mistakes are easy. One study demonstrated that a large proportion of insulin doses drawn up by people with diabetes, nurses and doctors were inaccurate. This is another reason for using an insulin pen. If you are doubtful about the accuracy of a particular dose discard it and start again. A small air bubble can cause a major inaccuracy, especially with small insulin doses.

It helps gently to rotate cloudy insulin bottles between your hands. But do not shake the bottle – the resultant froth takes a long time to settle. Cloudy insulin straight from the fridge may seem a little 'sticky'. New syringe plungers should be depressed fully before

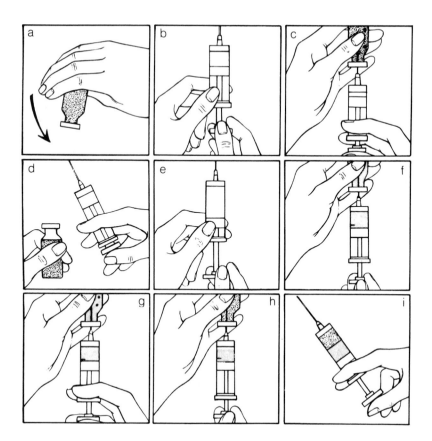

a) Gently rotate bottle to mix insulin
b) Draw up air
c) Inject air into cloudy insulin bottle
d) Put cloudy insulin down
e) Draw up air
f) Inject air into clear insulin bottle. Draw up clear insulin
g) Express air bubbles and check you have drawn up correct dose of clear insulin
h) Draw up correct dose of cloudy insulin
i) Ready for injection

Drying up and mixing insulin

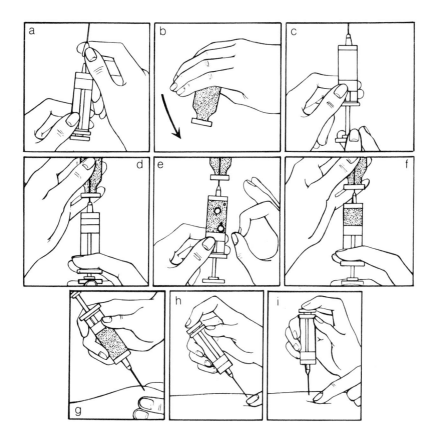

a) Attach needle to syringe if necessary
b) Gently rotate bottle to mix insulin
c) Draw up air and inject into the insulin bottle
d) Draw up insulin
e) Clear air bubbles
 f) Check syringe contains correct insulin dose
g) Inject insulin into fatty layer under skin
h) Withdraw needle
 i) Press on the hole

Injecting insulin

attempting to draw up insulin. Working the syringe plunger up and down vigorously is not necessary and can cause tiny fragments of rubber to come off.

Most problems seem to arise with mixing insulins. Now that so many fixed proportion insulins are available there is less need to mix. If you are mixing your own remember that you must *never* get cloudy insulin into your clear bottle. If you make an error discard that insulin and try again. Also remember that the only stable mixtures are those between clear insulin and cloudy isophane insulins. Other longer-acting insulins will start to convert your clear insulin to cloudy in the syringe and this will obviously alter its onset and duration of action. Always inject such a mixture immediately.

INJECTING YOUR INSULIN

Where

Inject insulin under the skin (subcutaneously). If you inject it into the skin surface you will get painful, white, firm blisters which leave red spots. If you inject it too deeply so the needle enters the muscles it may be painful and the insulin will be absorbed too quickly. Most of your subcutaneous tissue is fat with little blood vessels running through it. They will carry the insulin away gradually. Take a good pinch of skin and subcutaneous tissue and slide your needle in at an angle.

> Ali is a young athlete who trains hard every day. When he became diabetic he found it very difficult to inject his insulin because he had so little subcutaneous tissue. His glucose kept falling precipitously within an hour of his injection because he had injected the insulin into the muscle. Eventually he devised a technique whereby he pinched up the skin firmly and put the needle in virtually horizontally with the syringe lying close to his body.

The best places to inject insulin are the top of the thighs, upper buttocks, abdomen (tummy), and upper arms. You can also use your 'spare tyre' if you have one. A few people use their calves but this requires careful technique to avoid intramuscular injection and should not be used if you have poor circulation or varicose veins. Use as much of your chosen area as possible. Do not overuse any part of an injection site.

> Augustus was 75 and had had insulin-treated diabetes for 20 years.

94

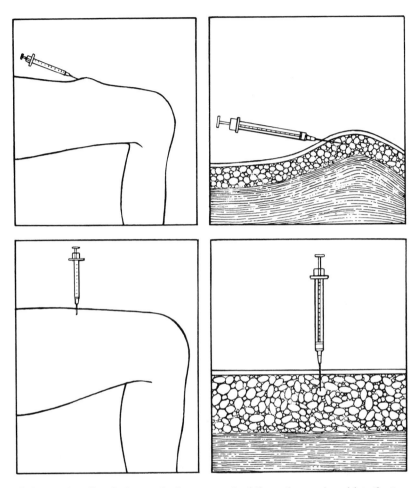

Injecting insulin. Only use the bottom method if you have a lot of fat; the top method is safest.

He rarely came to diabetic clinic and usually refused examination when he did come. One winter he was admitted to hospital with pneumonia. The doctor who admitted him was horrified to discover a black hole on the front of each thigh. 'That's where I puts me insulin' said Augustus.

A less dramatic consequence of overusing a particular site is lumps or dents. The lumps are called insulin hypertrophy and the dents insulin atrophy. Insulin absorption from these sites will be erratic. If you have an area like this change your injection site.

Many factors can affect the rate and amount of insulin absorption. Insulin is absorbed fastest from the arms, then the abdomen, then the legs, then the buttocks. However, if you increase the circulation to the injection site by warming it (by sun-bathing or sitting in a hot bath, for example) or by exercising the muscle underneath (by running, for example), your insulin will be absorbed faster than usual and your blood glucose may fall unexpectedly. If the injection site gets cold (outside in winter, for example) the insulin will be absorbed very slowly – until you warm up and then it may be absorbed quickly and when you are not expecting it. Cigarette smoking causes erratic insulin absorption because of the adverse effect of nicotine on the circulation. This means that the same dose of insulin in the same site may be absorbed at a different rate on Monday (football), Tuesday (sauna), Wednesday (sitting watching television) and Thursday (stopped smoking).

How

There is no need to clean your skin unless it is very dirty – and you should have daily all-over washes if you have diabetes. Spirit or alcohol harden the skin and cause stinging injections. However, if possible, you should wash your hands before drawing up and injecting. Pinch up the skin and subcutaneous tissue with one hand, hold your pen or syringe with the other and quickly put the needle through the skin. When you are sure that the needle tip is in the subcutaneous layer push down the plunger or twist the pen top to inject your insulin steadily, count to three, and quickly withdraw the needle. Put your finger firmly over the hole. Do not worry if you see a little blood, it is from a tiny vessel and will soon stop. Quick firm injections are less likely to sting than a slow tentative approach. Practise on an orange first using a spare syringe and needle with some water.

What happens now?

You eat. Once you have injected the insulin you cannot 'get it back'. It will be absorbed and will lower your blood glucose. It is therefore important that you eat after injecting all insulins except the very gentle long-acting bedtime ones. However, you should not fall into the old trap of adapting your meals to suit your insulin. This limits you and there is no reason why you should not adjust your insulin to suit your meal plans. Ask your diabetes adviser how to do this. If your meals are very erratic, a pre-meal pen insulin pattern may suit you best.

ADJUSTING YOUR INSULIN

Once you are confident about insulin injections and understand how each of your insulins affects you, you can learn to adjust your own treatment. There are several commonsense rules. At first, decide what you think you should do and then telephone your diabetes adviser to check that you have got it right. Gradually you will be able to sort it out yourself. Alter only one insulin in any one day unless your blood glucose level is very high or very low. Alter your insulin by only one or two units at first until you become more confident. Remember that if you increase your insulin there is a small risk of hypoglycaemia and be especially alert for this. Each change in your cloudy insulin dose will take about three days to settle down. So it is not a good idea to alter cloudy insulins more often than once every three days. You can alter your clear insulin each day if necessary. Never stop your insulin.

Some practical problems and what to do

Cracked or broken insulin bottle Throw it away – you must have at least one spare bottle of each sort of insulin.

Bent needles You are not keeping it in a straight line with the bottle while drawing up or injecting. Try to keep your hands steady.

Syringe jams Throw it away. Syringes may jam if you work the plunger vigorously – there is no need to do this. Sometimes happens with Ultratard insulin, especially if it is cold. Wait until the insulin is at room temperature. If you still have problems contact your diabetes adviser.

Painful injection Too deep or too shallow. Wrong angle, needle pulling on skin. Wet alcohol or other cleanser on the skin. Let it dry or do not use it. Too slow or jerky. Tender area – try somewhere else.

Spots at injection sites Too shallow. Skin irritated by cleanser. Very tender, red, swollen spot may be an infection – very rare. See your doctor that day.

ESSENTIAL EMERGENCY INFORMATION

Low blood glucose or hypoglycaemia

If you have too much insulin for your current needs your blood glucose will fall below normal (i.e. less than 4 mmol/1, or 72 mg/dl). You will become hypoglycaemic. This is rarely dramatic or severe and in the vast majority of episodes you will realise that your glucose is falling long before you feel more than slightly off-colour. However, you must be prepared for this. This means that from your first insulin injection and as long as you continue on insulin you must carry glucose or some other sugar on your person at all times and have it by you at night. You must also carry a diabetic card so that others could help you in the very unlikely event of your needing assistance.

Read about hypoglycaemia in Chapter 10. For practical purposes if you feel odd or unwell in any way check your glucose. If you find checking your glucose at all difficult, stop and eat some glucose immediately.

Because it takes a few days or weeks to establish a pattern of insulin treatment to suit you, you are at increased risk of hypoglycaemia during this time. DO NOT drive a car, operate machinery, work at heights, or take responsibility for other people's lives (e.g. carry a small baby, work as a nurse) for a week after starting insulin or beginning a new pattern of insulin treatment or a new type of insulin. Discuss the exact safety period with your diabetes adviser.

High blood glucose or hyperglycaemia

Few people with diabetes have normal blood glucose levels all the time. Each person should discuss high blood glucose levels with his or her diabetes adviser before it becomes a problem. These are very general guidelines and there is more detail in Chapter 11. Blood glucose levels always in double figures – i.e. 10 mmol/l or more (180 mg/dl or more) – are unacceptable and you should work to reduce them. It is not always easy so do not demand too much of yourself. If your blood glucose is over 19 mmol/l, you must do something about it now.

One high glucose If you know it is due to overeating, take 1–4 units of extra clear insulin to cover that meal and plan better next time (i.e. don't eat so much or have more insulin before the meal). Check your glucose again in two to four hours. If you feel well and the repeat glucose is under 19 mmol/l, do not worry.

A rising glucose but feeling well If the glucose is persistently high it means that your insulin dose is not covering what you are eating and your body housekeeping. If you are overweight consider eating less. If not, increase your insulin according to blood glucose; try 1–4 units of whichever insulin acts at that time of day. Check your urine for ketones. Contact your diabetes adviser within 48 hours. If more than a trace of ketones (i.e. more than one plus) are present contact your diabetes adviser that day.

A rising glucose and feeling ill This is an emergency. Continue your usual insulin and if your glucose is 19 mmol/l or more (342 mg/dl or more), give yourself 4–8 extra units of insulin (or the dose your diabetes adviser has advised in your teaching sessions) and contact your doctor immediately. He should see you that day. Continue to measure your glucose every two to four hours and write the results down. Check your urine for ketones. If there is more than one plus of ketones you are markedly insulin deficient. While these urine ketones persist give yourself 2–8 extra units of insulin (preferably fast-acting) every four hours if your glucose remains above 19 mmol/l. Do not forget to give your usual insulin as well.

If you become too ill to check your own blood glucose you need to be in hospital now. Call an ambulance by dialling 999 in the UK or the emergency number of the country you are in.

If your breathing becomes deep and sighing and you have urinary ketones, you must be in hospital whatever your blood glucose. You have ketoacidosis. Call an ambulance.

If you are vomiting (with or without raised blood glucose levels) you need to see a doctor within the next few hours – call one. If you have any problems contacting a doctor go to hospital.

NEVER STOP YOUR INSULIN

You need insulin to survive. If you stop taking it you will become acutely insulin deficient. Ketones will build up in your blood and you may become comatose. Even if you have a hypoglycaemic episode you should not stop your insulin. Eat glucose and more food, and, if necessary, reduce the dose. Contact your diabetes adviser for help. But do not stop it.

If you stop your insulin because you are vomiting from gastro-enteritis or some other infectious illness you will be cutting off your insulin at a time when your blood glucose levels are rising in response to the infection. This is a recipe for disaster. You will become very ill, very quickly. Occasionally diabetics encounter doctors not familiar with insulin-treated diabetes who try to stop their insulin. This situation can be difficult to handle. Explain politely that you have been told never to stop your insulin – and why. Show them this book. Suggest they contact your diabetes adviser.

Most people do not have dramatic problems with a minor bout of gastroenteritis. However, it can be hard to handle if you are newly insulin-treated which is why you need immediate advice. Often you will get better at home with fluids and more insulin. Otherwise fluids and insulin into a vein in hospital will soon solve the problem. Do not be afraid to ask the hospital for help. But in most instances you will be able to manage at home.

SUMMARY

- If your body cannot make insulin you must give it by injection.
- Find the insulin injection method and pattern which suits you.
- Clear insulins work fast. Cloudy insulins work slowly.
- Learn how to adjust your insulin according to your blood glucose measurements.
- Learn how to adjust your insulin according to your blood glucose measurements.
- Look after your insulin and equipment.
- Know who to contact for help.
- Always keep a back-up supply of insulin and needles and syringes.
- Pay attention to detail when drawing up your dose of insulin and injecting it. Get it right.
- Remember the variability of insulin absorption from injection sites.
- Always carry your diabetic card.
- Always carry glucose.
- Beware hypoglycaemia.
- Plan what to do if your glucose rises or you become ill.
- Vomiting is a danger sign. Heed it.
- Remember, tailor your insulin treatment to suit your needs.
- Never stop your insulin.

10

HYPOGLYCAEMIA OR LOW BLOOD GLUCOSE

If you are taking pills or insulin to lower your blood glucose you must read this chapter carefully. Hypoglycaemia is rarely a major problem but it is common and you must learn to recognise its earliest symptoms and act on them promptly.

HYPOGLYCAEMIA: BACKGROUND INFORMATION

How common is hypoglycaemia?

An insulin-treated diabetic can expect about 10 hypoglycaemic episodes each year. About one in three people on insulin will need treatment for hypoglycaemia from someone else each year. In other words, each year you have a one in three chance that you will have an episode that you have difficulty treating on your own. Learning how to recognise your early warnings and taking prompt action will reduce this risk. People with diabetes taking glucose-lowering pills are less likely to become hypoglycaemic but it can occur and you too must be able to recognise the symptoms. It may take you longer to get your glucose back to normal should you become hypoglycaemic.

How can you prevent problems with hypoglycaemia?

Firstly, by keeping a close eye on your blood glucose and planning ahead – more of this later in the chapter. Secondly, by learning to recognise all of your own hypoglycaemia symptoms, however minor, so that you can treat them immediately. I believe that people with diabetes are better at recognising their own hypoglycaemia than they realise. Hypoglycaemia may actually make you forget what happened, but you can sometimes write symptoms down at the time – once you have eaten your glucose, of course. Have a high index of suspicion; if you are new to insulin ask yourself if every unusual feeling may be due to a low glucose. As I write this I can almost hear diabetes advisers who read this saying 'She'll turn them all into terrified neurotics, thinking every itch and sniff is a hypo and afraid to do anything in case they go hypo'. Oh no, I won't! My readers have more common sense than that. You must control your diabetes if you are to get on with enjoying life as you want it. To control your diabetes you must have the power to rule it. In knowledge lies power. Once you have learned your early warning clues you can treat an early hypoglycaemic attack with a quick mouthful of glucose tablets and carry on. You will not have to wait until it gets so bad you have difficulty in managing it yourself.

What is hypoglycaemia?

There is no generally accepted definition of hypoglycaemia, although most would accept a laboratory venous blood glucose below 2.5 mmol/l as indisputably hypoglycaemic. For practical purposes, in a person with diabetes on glucose-lowering treatment, it is a finger-prick blood glucose level below 4 mmol/l (72 mg/dl), with or without symptoms; or symptoms or signs substantially and rapidly improved by giving glucose, sucrose or glucagon (see below).

SYMPTOMS OF HYPOGLYCAEMIA

These are usually divided into two sorts. Firstly, those due to the brain being deprived of its main fuel, glucose. Medspeak for these is 'neuroglycopaenic symptoms'. Secondly, those due to the body's emergency response. Medspeak for these is 'adrenergic symptoms'. In practice, the symptoms of hypoglycaemia for any one person do not necessarily fit the classical pattern. Each person must learn to recognise his or her own symptoms as early as possible.

Problems with thinking and awareness

These may be very early signs. Lack of concentration should lead you to suspect that you are hypoglycaemic. You may find yourself taking a very long time to do a simple sum or unable to understand a newspaper article. You may be unable to make decisions – simple ones like 'Shall I have tea or coffee?'. You may start to become muddled or find that your thoughts or what people say does not make sense. You may not be able to find the right words, or you may start to talk and talk. You may become very confused and get lost, or be unable to finish a task. Your eyes may feel heavier and heavier until you fall asleep.

Not wanting to eat

One part of your brain may tell you that you need food while another says 'Yeucch!' and refuses. Hopefully the first part will win.

'I've started so I'll finish'

One common feeling is that you must complete the task you were engaged in as your glucose started to fall. If you are driving a car this inner voice telling you to drive on must be resisted at all costs. Stop immediately you suspect you may be hypoglycaemic. I once watched a hypoglycaemic man trying to get an apple from a polythene bag. Despite my holding glucose tablets out to him he insisted on opening the bag. It kept slipping in his sweaty fingers. In the end I stuffed the glucose into his mouth and as he came to he allowed me to open the bag and hand him an apple.

Emotions

Quiet people may feel like being noisy and vice versa. You may feel extraordinarily happy or giggly – everything is a huge joke. Or you may feel very sad – everything is low and miserable. Quite often people who are hypoglycaemic get cross. You may become irritable because you cannot calculate your change in a shop, or shout at your wife because she asks what you want for dinner and you cannot decide. Or you may become furious with everyone for no particular reason. You may feel that everyone is against you – and this feeling may be worsened by people's attempts to help you to get better. (Carers should, however, remember that people with diabetes have the same emotions as everyone else. Nothing is more infuriating than people saying 'There, there, you're not really cross, you're hypo, have some glucose, dear' when the person is genuinely angry and not in the least hypoglycaemic.)

Problems with movement and co-ordination

Co-ordination skills are often reduced early in hypoglycaemia. You may feel very clumsy – buttons won't do up, you cannot open your packet of glucose tablets. You drop things. You may start staggering and eventually be unable to walk. Your arms and legs may not work properly and, rarely, you may be unable to move part of your body.

Weakness or superhuman strength

You might expect that lack of fuel would make your whole body weak and this is often the case. You may feel as if you are wading through porridge. However, occasionally people briefly become extremely strong and can run or fight. You may feel invincible.

Altered vision

Blurring of vision sometimes occurs. Or you may see the world with abnormal clarity – as if it is new and wonderful. One of my friends said that the sky always turned pink when he became hypoglycaemic.

Palpitations

This means increased awareness of unusually rapid heart beats. It can occur as the glucose is falling.

Sweating

Torrential sweating which soaks your clothes is a clear sign of hypoglycaemia. However, it may be quite a late sign and occur only as the glucose is rising again.

Trembling

This is a fine shaking of your hands but it may add to the problems of inco-ordination, making it difficult for you to take glucose.

Anything else

There is a huge variety of symptoms of hypoglycaemia; some seem unique to one person. Any unusual sensation should be assumed to be due to hypoglycaemia until proved otherwise.

SIGNS OF HYPOGLYCAEMIA

These are for carers to note – although some may be apparent to the hypoglycaemic person.

Not himself or herself

The early signs may be very subtle and apparent only to someone who knows the person well. Very small changes which you cannot pin-point but which make you vaguely uneasy or look twice may indicate hypoglycaemia. Look three times.

Problems with thinking or alertness

The lack of concentration may be more apparent to you than to the sufferers themselves. Their thoughts and movements may be painfully slow. I have learnt that when a patient in diabetic clinic is taking an inordinately long time to understand or answer what seem to be simple questions he or she is nearly always hypoglycaemic. It may be hard to keep such patients to the point and they may not appear able to obey simple instructions. Undue sleepiness in the day or difficulty waking someone in the morning is another sign.

Emotions

This is probably one of the factors in the 'not himself' sign. But more obvious emotional changes often appear. Undue quietness in the 'life-and-soul of the party'. Extrovert behaviour from an introvert. Irritability and a desire to be left alone is common. 'I don't want help. I'm not hypo. Go away.' People with diabetes will be annoyed to read the next bit but it is something I have learned the hard way. If someone on insulin says that they are definitely not hypoglycaemic, especially if they are very cross or fed up when they say it, their glucose is often falling fast (but see page 103).

Teresa McLean in her book *Metal Jam* said 'Although a part of my brain often knows that I am feeling hypo, the state itself stops me being able to do anything about it. Nor am I able to admit my problem to anyone I am with. If asked, I always deny that anything is wrong. It is this inability to explain to others that I need sugar once a hypo has started which baffles everyone around me.'

Marion was returning from a long mountain walk. She was stumbling and seemed likely to fall. We asked if she thought she might be hypoglycaemic. 'I'm not hypo. Of course I'm not hypo.

How could anyone who was hypo do this?' And before we could stop her she had climbed a rock and was balancing on one leg, other leg outstretched with toe pointed balletically. When we retrieved her, Marion's finger prick blood glucose was 2 mmol/l.

Sometimes people with hypoglycaemia may think that people trying to help them are attacking them and resist with all their force – I was hurt by a hypoglycaemic 80 year old. She also injured two ambulancemen, a nurse, and a large, rugby-playing medical student.

Problems with movement and co-ordination

Clumsiness or stumbling combined with inco-ordination, slurred speech and confusion can make a markedly hypoglycaemic person appear drunk. However, such gross problems are uncommon and you must watch for smaller difficulties – dropping a cup while washing up or stubbing a toe on a paving stone perhaps. I have noticed that hypoglycaemic people may bump into you while walking beside you. Rarely it can seem as if someone with hypoglycaemia is having a stroke, but in this case glucose will restore completely normal function within minutes.

Inappropriate or unusual behaviour

Rarely, severe hypoglycaemia can make people do odd things – sunbathe on a windowsill in the evening, attack people with a brush, unpack something they have just packed. They may talk nonsense or run up a hill they have just walked down. Or simply stand and smile without moving. Don't laugh. Treat the hypoglycaemia.

Fast pulse, pallor, trembling and sweating

The shakiness and sweating will be obvious. Feel the pulse – it is usually fast (say 100 beats per minute rather than 70). The skin may become very pale, or occasionally flushed, sometimes patchily.

Coma and fits

Although first aid books may give the impression that all hypogly-caemia is coma this is not true. Coma or lack of consciousness is rare in hypoglycaemia. Sometimes people who are unconscious from hypoglycaemia have a convulsive fit. This may appear frightening but both the coma and the fits are immediately relieved by glucose.

DON'T PANIC

By now both those of you with diabetes and your carers and family may be worried. No-one has all these features and most people never have dramatic changes with hypoglycaemia. Coma is rare. I have collected these signs and symptoms from thousands of people with diabetes seen over many years. Furthermore, hypoglycaemia is one of the most wonderful medical conditions to treat – give glucose, the patient recovers in minutes and is soon his or her usual self again.

TREATMENT OF HYPOGLYCAEMIA

Test your glucose if you can

If the symptoms are minimal and you are in a safe situation, test your blood glucose and confirm that you are indeed hypoglycaemic. If you are, eat some glucose. If you find any aspect of blood testing difficult abandon it and eat glucose.

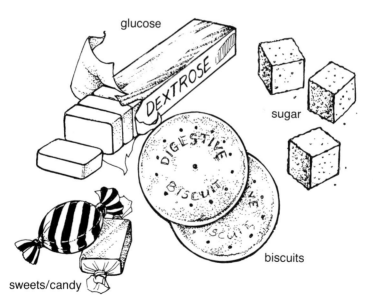

Foods to be consumed for treatment of hypoglycaemia

Eat glucose or sucrose

The best emergency treatment for a low blood glucose is glucose. It will be absorbed most quickly in liquid form – for example as a glucose drink such as Lucozade. However, this may not be convenient to carry around. Glucose tablets (Boots, Dextrosol, Lucozade and others) are simplest. Try to wash them down with water or another drink, if possible. There are also sweets which contain glucose. Sucrose, as sugar lumps or in sweets or candies also work quickly, but the sucrose has to be digested to glucose before absorption.

For water sports, Hypostop glucose gel is easier. It is in a leakproof plastic bottle which you can put in a pocket in a swimming costume or boating gear.

If you are unable to feed yourself your friends or relatives may have to post glucose tablets into your mouth. Firm, direct command is best. 'Eat this now. No, don't spit it out. Eat it now.' Again, a glucose drink may be quicker. Some people insist on a particular food to cure their hypoglycaemia – like a Mars Bar or, in the case of an elderly lady who became hypoglycaemic in Diabetic Clinic, a strawberry jam sandwich.

Eat food

The elderly lady was partly right. Once you have eaten or drunk your glucose, have something more substantial to keep your blood glucose up. A sandwich, a couple of digestive biscuits, a bowl of muesli or a muesli bar. If you do not eat something solid and you still have too much insulin in your circulation, it will use up all the glucose you have just eaten and you will become hypoglycaemic again.

Glucagon

Partners and relatives of insulin-treated diabetics should always have glucagon in the house. This is rarely necessary if you are taking glucose-lowering pills. Take glucagon with you when you are travelling. It is the hormone which works opposite to insulin – it raises the blood glucose by releasing it from the liver stores. Unlike insulin it is not stable in solution and comes in a pack containing a bottle of dry powder, and water with a syringe and needle. The pack must be in date.

Use glucagon if the hypoglycaemic person will not or cannot swallow. For example, if the person is so confused you cannot persuade him to eat glucose, or if he is unconscious. If you need the glucagon, do not rush. First put an unconscious person in the recovery position (see below). Get the box out, hold it and take a deep breath in and out (to calm yourself). Then open the box carefully. Draw up the water into the syringe (some syringes are pre-filled with water) and squirt it into the bottle containing the powder. Mix gently. Then draw back all the solution into the syringe and hold it needle up. If there are air bubbles tap up to the top and squirt them out. Then inject the glucagon deep into the big muscles in the side of the thigh. It does not matter if some goes subcutaneously, nor if it enters a vein, provided there are no air bubbles. If the person is fighting you or you cannot undress him, inject through the trousers. This technique is only to be used in dire emergencies. Injections through clothes, even tights, carry the risk of introducing bits of fibre under the skin which can act as a focus for infection.

Glucagon has a temporary effect only. Once the person is awake and rational you must feed him. This may be difficult because glucagon makes some people feel sick and 'hungover'.

Coma and fits

The main danger is not that of the low blood glucose but of the unconsciousness itself. You must protect the airway before you do anything else. Check that there is nothing in the mouth. Then roll the person onto his side, being careful to keep the mouth away from the floor. The illustration shows the recovery position in which it is safe to leave the patient while you get the glucagon or call for help. Otherwise you must not leave him unattended until he has woken up. If he is having a fit move all the furniture away so that he cannot injure himself and keep him on his side. Do not attempt to force anything into his mouth. The tongue is bitten in the first instant of the fit and you will only cause further injury – to the patient and perhaps, to yourself.

Once you have injected the glucagon, keep the person on his side and wait. He will wake up within a quarter of an hour. If he does not, immediately phone an ambulance. Phone your doctor or an ambulance in any case if you are at all worried. The doctor can always wake the person up by injecting concentrated glucose into a vein.

While it is dangerous to give anything by mouth to someone who is unconscious in case they inhale it, years of experience, especially with children, has shown that small amounts of glucose rubbed inside the cheek or gums, may help to rouse them. Small amounts of Hypostop can be used in this way. Always lie the patient on his side with his airway clear and watch that you do not get bitten fingers.

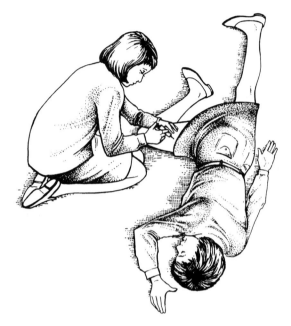

Recovery position and injecting glucagon

WHY WERE YOU HYPOGLYCAEMIC?

As soon as you feel better work out why you became hypoglycaemic. The main causes are:

- Too much insulin or too many glucose-lowering pills;
- Not enough food;
- Unexpected or strenuous exercise.

Too much insulin or too many glucose-lowering pills

Everyone is capable of making mistakes – did you take more insulin or pills than you intended? Did you inject the insulin more deeply than usual so that it entered the muscle? Is your insulin dose too big – look back over your previous blood glucose tests and see whether you often have lower readings at this time. Is your pill dosage too high? Check the label on the bottle.

Not enough food

This is a common reason for hypoglycaemia. Did you miss a meal because you were in a hurry or did not like it? Were the portions smaller than expected? The wise person with diabetes has a muesli bar or biscuits in a bag, briefcase or pocket to ensure that she has something to eat at any time. Dieting to lose weight without first reducing your dose of insulin or glucose-lowering pills is another reason for frequent hypoglycaemia (especially in weight-conscious young women).

Unexpected or strenuous exercise

Running for a bus, playing an expected game of tennis, finding a tough job in the garden, unloading a lorry that you were not expecting; exertion like this can lower your blood glucose fast. Eat extra glucose while you are exercising. Note that I said unexpected exercise – if you know you are going to exercise you should plan ahead (see Chapter 17).

HYPOGLYCAEMIC UNAWARENESS

After many years of diabetes about one in five people lose awareness of some or all their symptoms of hypoglycaemia. About one in 15 have no warning symptoms at all. This appears to be related to long duration of diabetes, and, in some cases, to diabetic autonomic nerve damage (see page 139). Beta blocker pills used to treat high blood pressure or angina (see pages 129 and 140) can diminish your warning of hypoglycaemia. Never stop these pills without first consulting your doctor.

Human insulin

There has been some anxiety that human insulins are more likely to cause problems with hypoglycaemia than animal insulins. Human insulin was introduced at a time when there was also increasing encouragement to keep blood glucose concentrations as close to normal as possible. This strategy is to protect people from long-term tissue damage but it does mean that there is more risk of hypoglycaemia and less warning. It usually takes less time for the glucose to fall from 5 to 2 mmol/l (90–36 mg/dl), than to fall from 12 to 2 mmol/l (216–36 mg/dl). Insulin-treated diabetics with persistently normal blood glucose levels have less emergency hormone response to hypoglycaemia than those who usually have high blood glucose

111

levels. One survey (around the time of some media publicity against human insulin) asked people to remember what their hypo-glycaemia was like before and after starting human insulin. One in twelve of those who had warning of hypoglycaemia before the changeover said they had less warning since – but one in 24 had more warning – and, of course all of them had another few years of diabetes. If you have had diabetes for long enough to remember taking animal insulin you may have diabetic tissue damage which, among other effects, can reduce your warning of hypoglycaemia. A study in Switzerland showed that people requiring hospital treatment for severe hypoglycaemia were more likely to be taking human insulin than patients with diabetes admitted for other reasons. However, those admitted for hypoglycaemia also had better blood glucose control than the others. Another Swiss study compared human with pork insulin in 44 people. Each person took both, but neither patients nor doctors knew which insulin was being taken. A blood glucose below 2.8 mmol/l was recorded more often when they were taking the pork insulin. While taking human insulin, hypoglycaemic people were more likely to report restlessness and lack of concentration and less likely to report hunger than during hypoglycaemia on pork insulin. A British survey of about 6000 insulin-treated people found just 19 people who reported loss of warning of hypoglycaemia for which the only reason seemed to be taking human insulin, and who regained their warning symptoms on restarting animal insulin. Seven of them agreed to be made hypoglycaemic with either pork or human insulin under identical conditions without knowing which insulin they were receiving. There was no difference in their feelings, their blood glucose, or in their emergency hormone response to either insulin.

At the time of writing, if I had diabetes I personally would want human insulin treatment. However, if you feel that you had better warning of hypoglycaemia on animal insulin, or you have any other concerns about human insulin, discuss it with your doctor and, if you are still unhappy, ask to change to animal insulin. You may not be able to have insulin with exactly the same duration and pattern of action as your human one(s) and you will not be able to use a pen as there are no animal insulin cartridges. Time will hopefully clarify the issue, but it is essential that you have confidence in your treatment now.

Watch your blood glucose

I am always a little surprised when people show me their blood glucose diaries with 2s (36 mg/dl) dotted about and then say that they have had no hypos since I last saw them. When I point to the 2s they say that they did not feel hypo then. Whether or not you feel hypoglycaemic, a blood glucose of 2 mmol/l (36 mg/dl) is hypoglycaemic and requires immediate treatment and then review as to why it happened. So if the result is 2, STOP, eat.

Some people are fine during the day but their blood glucose dips at night. You may detect this by waking feeling hungover or with a headache. If you are on insulin make sure you always have a bed-time snack and do not go to bed with a glucose below 6 mmol/l (108 mg/dl). It is sensible to set an alarm clock for 2 or 3 am from time to time to check your blood glucose level.

> Tracey was 17. She wanted to learn how to drive. I asked how her diabetes was. 'Good,' she said, 'I've been really careful'. I asked to see her diabetic diary. All the blood glucose levels were 4 or below. At least half were 2 mmol/l or less. I was horrified. She admitted she did feel low quite often. She was very upset when I said that she was not safe to drive. After she had calmed down and we discussed it all, it emerged that she thought a previous doctor had told her to keep her blood glucose levels as low as possible to avoid tissue damage. She had been doing exactly as she was told. We reduced her insulin dose and her blood glucose concentrations became normal. She passed her driving test a year later.

HONEYMOON PERIOD

In the weeks or months after starting insulin treatment your few remaining islet cells, which had been 'stunned' by the high glucose levels, may start making insulin again. You may become hypoglycaemic and your insulin requirements may plummet. This is called the honeymoon period. Eventually these cells will succumb to the auto-immune process and die. You will need bigger insulin doses again.

SUMMARY

- Hypoglycaemia is a low blood glucose – below 4 mmol/l for practical purposes, official definition below 2.5 mmol/l.
- It is common in insulin-treated diabetics (about 10 episodes a

year) and occurs in one in three people who are taking gliben-clamide.

- Hypoglycaemia is rarely serious.
- Learn to recognise when your blood glucose is falling.
- Teach your friends and family what to look for.
- Always carry glucose if you take insulin or sulphonylurea pills.
- Eat glucose immediately you become hypoglycaemic, followed by some starchy food.
- When you are better work out why you were hypoglycaemic. Was it too much insulin or too many pills, too little food, or unexpected exercise?
- Bad hypos are rare. If you are on insulin keep glucagon in the house just in case.
- Good observation and early treatment of hypoglycaemia can prevent trouble.

11

HYPERGLYCAEMIA OR HIGH BLOOD GLUCOSE

In theory, any blood glucose over 8 mmol/l (144 mg/dl) is high, i.e. hyperglycaemic. However, while everyone would like to have their blood glucose levels between 4 and 8 mmol/l (72–144 mg/dl), in real life it is very hard to achieve this all the time over years of diabetes. That does not mean that you should stop trying.

For practical purposes, this chapter is about blood glucose levels in double figures (i.e. 11 mmol/l or more – 200 mg/dl USA). Many of you will see blood glucose levels in this range from time to time; the occasional level between 11 and 20 mmol/l is rarely a disaster although it may make you feel below par, thirsty or pass a lot of urine.

One of the difficulties in advising people with diabetes about how to respond to changes in blood glucose is that everyone responds differently to a given blood glucose. Some people who do not look after their diabetes walk around with blood glucose levels of 30 mmol/l (540 mg/dl) and claim to feel fine. Others feel awful if their glucose rises about 11 mmol/l (200 mg/dl). Part of this is due to the body getting used to the prevailing glucose level, but we all perceive things differently. In addition other factors, such as the state of other body chemistry, will affect how you feel and how seriously to take a particular glucose level. This makes it hard to use particular blood glucose levels to indicate particular courses of action. Each of you must get to know your own body. Discuss with your diabetes adviser what you are going to do if your glucose rises – what follows is general guidance only.

PERSISTENTLY HIGH BLOOD GLUCOSE LEVELS

11–19 mmol/l (200–342 mg/dl)

Sadly, many people with diabetes have levels like this most of the time. Part of this may be a legacy of the days when you were told, 'Always keep a little sugar in your urine to stop you going hypo'. If there is glucose in the urine your blood glucose is likely to be over 11 mmol/l. The threshold for the development of some diabetic complications appears to be about 11–12 mmol/l (200–216 mg/dl). This means that if your average blood glucose is above this for long periods of time, you may develop diabetic tissue damage (see Chapter 12).

Thus, while for most people these blood glucose levels are not acutely dangerous, they may be slowly harming your body and should be reduced.

Over 19 mmol/l (342–mg/dl)

Most people with insulin-treated diabetes will have one-off levels like this at some time. However, if most of your blood glucose levels are this high you are in danger. Although you may not feel very ill, a small upset – a row at work, or a cold, for example – could push your blood glucose up fast. Then you could feel very ill. Levels like this require immediate action.

SOME CAUSES OF A HIGH BLOOD GLUCOSE

- Too little insulin or glucose-lowering pills;
- Too much food;
- Too little exercise;
- Monthly periods;
- Pregnancy;
- Infection;
- Injury or operation;
- Heart attack;
- Stress;
- Drugs and medicines.

Too little insulin or too few glucose-lowering pills

If you forget your insulin, run out or stop taking it, your glucose will

116

rise. If you forget your diabetic pills, run out or stop taking them, your glucose will rise. Glucose-lowering treatments are your lifeline – by all means reduce your treatment if your blood glucose is persistently low (see Chapter 10), but do not stop it. There is no excuse for running out of pills and to run out of insulin is unforgivable. The occasional forgotten dose is human, but if you keep forgetting develop a system for remembering – an alarm clock beside the insulin if necessary. Do not stop your insulin during a vomiting illness.

Too much food

Lucy was an in-patient on the diabetic ward. She had been admitted with pneumonia which upset her blood glucose balance. Although the pneumonia soon improved her blood glucose levels went up and up. Eventually we discovered that she was having two breakfasts – one on the ward and a second one in the staff canteen. 'I do like a cooked breakfast', she said, 'and I can't be bothered at home'. She liked the canteen's afternoon teas too.

If you eat more than the insulin in your body can cope with (whether your own insulin, that boosted by pills or injected insulin) then your blood glucose will rise. A few people need to put on weight if new diabetes has made them thin. In most cases extra weight is the last thing you need. As you get fat, your insulin needs rise, your insulin dose or pills must be increased, this makes you hungry, you eat more, and so on.

A few people try to starve their glucose down. This is not a good idea. It causes fat breakdown which makes ketones.

Too little exercise

Damian was in the sixth month of his first job. The job was going well but his diabetes wasn't. His blood glucose levels had started to rise soon after he began the job and he seemed to need more insulin these days. He could not understand it because he was sticking to his diet. He discussed it with Mrs Baxter, the Diabetes Specialist Nurse. 'How much exercise do you get these days?' she asked. 'Not much,' replied Damian, ruefully. 'I really enjoy all the planning work I do in the office, but I miss the school football team. No-one here seems interested in sport.' This was why his glucose levels had risen. His exercise level had dropped as soon as he left school. He was not burning off the glucose as he used to. When Mrs Baxter checked his weight that had increased a little. She suggested eating

117

a little less and using the factory swimming pool several times a week to keep fit. There he met several sportsmen and was soon playing squash regularly.

Regular exercise increases your sensitivity to insulin and improves the way in which you use glucose. It keeps you fit generally (see Chapter 17).

Monthly periods

The hormone changes which occur during a woman's menstrual cycle can have profound effects on blood glucose. Most diabetic women find that their blood glucose rises just before or as they lose blood. A few notice a tendency to hypoglycaemia then a rise in glucose. The changes last only a few days in most people and are often not severe enough to alter the insulin dose. However, some women adjust their insulin with every period. Find out what happens to your own glucose levels. Glucose levels may fall after the menopause.

Pregnancy

As the pregnancy progresses your insulin needs will increase. Some women may be taking twice as much insulin by the end of pregnancy as they were at the start (see Chapter 16).

Infection

Any infection can upset your diabetes: a cold, 'flu, viral sore throat, cystitis (urine infection), chest infection, gastroenteritis, thrush, an abscess and so on. The degree to which your blood glucose rises during an infection is not always in proportion to the severity of the infection. However, the glucose can rise very fast – for example overnight it may go from 8 to 22 mmol/l (144–396 mg/dl). The reason for the rise in glucose (sometimes despite vomiting or eating less) is the release of emergency hormones (e.g. steroids, adrenaline) to help your body fight the infection. They release glucose from the liver into the bloodstream. So you need more insulin when you have an infection. As the infection settles you will need to reduce your insulin dose again. People on diet treatment alone may find that they need extra help – glucose-lowering pills or insulin injections while the infection resolves. Those on pills may find that they need insulin temporarily. Your body cannot fight the infection if your blood glucose level is high. This prevents your soldiers – the white blood cells – from moving in to attack and engulf the bacteria. So a vicious circle may

118

ensue – infection, glucose rises, defence slows, infection worsens, glucose rises more and so on. Get help early on to treat the infection and do not allow your blood glucose to rise. This means injecting your usual dose of insulin even if you are unable to eat and giving extra insulin if your blood glucose levels are high. You need energy to get better so if you cannot eat try drinking Lucozade, Coke, Pepsi, fruit juice, milk or soup. Ice cream or yoghurt may be easy to eat. But *on no account* stop your insulin.

Injury or operation

The body responds to injury – a broken leg, for example, as it does to infection. As far as the body is concerned, an operation is a form of injury. Stress hormones are released to help you recover and these release glucose into the bloodstream. You may need to increase your insulin while recovering from major injury. If you have an operation and cannot eat for a while you will usually be given insulin and glucose into a vein. The doses will be adjusted according to blood glucose levels until you are eating again. Then your usual insulin or pills can be restarted. With a major injury or operation people on diet alone may sometimes need insulin at this time.

Heart attack

See page 130. A heart attack is another form of stress and injury, and again emergency hormones are released pushing the blood glucose up. Your blood glucose level should be returned towards normal, making sure that you cannot become hypoglycaemic at a time when your heart may be irritable.

Stress

I have used the word 'stress' to mean a situation which evokes an emergency response in the body. The stress of everyday life can cause adrenaline release which may push the blood glucose up.

Mike was the shop steward in a glass factory. There had been increasing friction between a particular manager and the workers in the plate glass plant. This came to a head one Friday when the manager accused a man of sloppy work. Mike had a fierce argument with the manager and both sides eventually retired angry with the dispute unsettled. Mike drove home in a temper. When he checked his blood glucose it had risen from 9 mmol/l (162 mg/dl) at lunchtime to 19 mmol/l (342 mg/dl) – the highest evening level he had seen for years. He took three extra units of fast-acting insulin and by bedtime the glucose was down to 11 mmol/l (200 mg/dl).

Drugs and medicines

I do not mean street drugs, although these can upset your blood glucose (among other things) and are dangerous. Medical drugs are a common cause of hyperglycaemia. Steroids produce the greatest rise in glucose and the dose of insulin or glucose-lowering pills can double during a course of steroid treatment. If the steroids are stopped abruptly, the glucose will fall suddenly. This is important for diabetic asthmatics who may need short courses of steroids. Other drugs which may increase the blood glucose concentration are thiazide diuretics (see page 141), oral contraceptive pills and sometimes tricyclic antidepressants (e.g. amitriptylline). Thiazides can usually be changed to another medication to control high blood pressure or alleviate ankle swelling. Steroids are essential treatment for most of the conditions in which they are used, so you will have to adjust your diabetes treatment to follow the glucose rise (and its fall when the steroid treatment finishes).

WHAT DO YOU DO ABOUT HIGH BLOOD GLUCOSE LEVELS?

If the high value comes as a complete surprise, wash your hands and repeat the test carefully. You may have had sticky fingers.

Emergency advice for high blood glucose levels is given on page 98. To adjust your insulin you need to know which insulin is acting (or rather, should be acting) at the times when the blood glucose is high, and how long it acts for. As cloudy insulins take a long time to clear from the body it is best to wait three days between each dosage adjustment. Over-rapid changes in medium or long-acting insulin may lead to exaggerated glucose fluctuations and hypoglycaemia. It is also easiest (at least to start with) to adjust only one insulin dose (i.e. morning only or evening only) at a time, to avoid confusion. If you are nervous about increasing your insulin do it in one unit steps. Check with your diabetes adviser. But do not simply sit and look at high blood glucose levels and do nothing.

People taking glucose lowering pills can also adjust their medication if blood glucose levels are persistently high. But you must check with your diabetes adviser first. Each pill has a maximum dose which must not be exceeded (unlike insulin where you have as much as your body needs). The maximum doses are shown on page 74 – but these may be lower in people with some medical problems, such as kidney impairment. Again leave three days in between each dosage adjustment.

SUMMARY

- If your blood glucose is in double figures, i.e. 11 mmol (200 mg/dl) or more, you are at risk of thirst and polyuria now.
- If your blood glucose remains in double figures you are at risk of tissue damage later.
- If you feel well but your blood glucose is rising take extra insulin and adjust your diet or treatment to prevent future high glucose levels.
- If you feel ill and your blood glucose is rising, especially if you have urinary ketones, take extra insulin and get help urgently.
- Vomiting is a danger sign in diabetes. Get help.
- Causes of a high blood glucose include too little insulin or glucose-lowering pills, too much food, too little exercise, monthly periods, pregnancy, infection, injury, heart attack, stress, drugs.

12

DIABETIC TISSUE DAMAGE

Diabetes is a multi-system disorder. In other words, it affects many parts or systems of the body. So far, I have concentrated on blood glucose balance. But other blood chemicals are also disturbed in diabetes. And more problems arise from damage to body tissues than are caused by ups and downs of blood glucose. Many people do not link their heart attack or poor vision to their diabetes – but they are connected. They are also potentially preventable if you take care of yourself from the beginning.

Diabetes tissue damage is traditionally divided into small blood vessel damage, such as that which occurs in eyes or kidneys; and large blood vessel damage, occurring in vessels supplying the heart and legs. But problems may be a combination of these and other factors. Also, classifications which seem obvious to doctors do not always reflect what people actually notice in themselves. I will therefore discuss the effects of diabetes as you may discover them and how your doctor may assess and treat you. This approach means that common and uncommon complications are mixed up. Don't panic. No-one will have all of them! And if you do find a problem, your diabetes team can help you. In Chapter 13 I will review possible causes of these effects and what you can do to prevent them.

I have described potential problems according to parts of the body, where you may find them, or the doctor examining you may find them.

SKIN

Infections

Minor skin infections These are common in diabetes, especially if the blood glucose is not well controlled. There may be boils or spots which will settle as the blood glucose settles. Occasionally boils develop into abscesses or carbuncles. These may need surgical incision and drainage, sometimes under a general anaesthetic. Rarely, a rash of purple-red spots up the legs indicates a spreading bacterial infection by staphylococcus aureus needing antibiotic therapy. More often purple or red marks on the legs are scars due to old knocks and scrapes.

Thrush This may develop in cracks and crevices of the skin – under breasts or in the groins, if you are overweight. This will respond to antifungal cream, control of high blood glucose and weight loss.

Diabetic dermopathy

Many people with long-standing diabetes develop red/brown or brown marks on the skin. These may occur at the site of minor injury or spontaneously. They may fade a little but can last many years. No treatment is needed and they are not serious.

Necrobiosis lipoidica diabeticorum

Necrobiosis lipoidica diabeticorum is a rare complication of diabetes, usually found in people whose blood glucose has been too high for a long time. It is a red-purple shiny dent in the skin, usually over the lower leg. It may settle slowly on its own. If not, steroid treatment is sometimes helpful and some doctors use nicotinic acid tablets. The condition itself is not dangerous but it is occasionally sore and women may want to hide it with tights or make-up.

Eruptive xanthomata

These are little fatty lumps which are found in people with very high levels of the blood fat, triglyceride. Such people may have fatty streaks in the creases of their hands too. Eruptive xanthomata are quite rare and are most often found on the upper limbs. People with these need to lower their triglyceride fast (see page 148).

HEAD AND NECK:

General appearance

Facial appearance While not strictly a complication of diabetes, the following changes may alert you to the existence of a hormonal cause for your diabetes which was perhaps not obvious initially. A very round moon-face, with rosy red cheeks and (in women) excess hair on the chin, upper lip and sides may indicate steroid hormone excess (whether taken as tablets or due to overproduction in the body). Coarsening of the skin, heavy brows, a large protruding jaw and increased spacing of the teeth may indicate growth hormone excess (acromegaly – a rare condition). A slim face with an anxious expression and staring eyes may indicate thryoid overactivity.

Pimples and boils Facial pimples and boils on the back of the neck can cause much distress especially if you are young. They usually improve with good blood glucose balance. Acne can be treated with good skin care and sometimes tetracycline or related antibiotics.

Muscle weakness Facial muscle weakness can be due to a stroke (usually including cheek and side of the mouth) or to damage to one of the nerves supplying the face in which it may be more localised. If the facial nerves are not working (either due to a stroke or to nerve damage), you may not be able to control your mouth and saliva or food may dribble out of that side (rather like the effects of a dental local anaesthetic). Nerve damage may prevent the eyelid from opening fully. Facial weakness usually improves gradually.

Gustatory sweating This describes the flushing and sweating on the face precipitated by eating in someone with diabetic autonomic nerve damage (see page 139). It is best to avoid highly spiced foods if you have this problem.

Eyes

Squint with double vision This is another sign of weak muscles because of nerve damage. It may come on quite suddenly with pain or aching around the eye. Again this can resolve with time, improvement usually starting within weeks, although it may take many months for full recovery. An eye patch may help.

Cataract Cataract is common in people with diabetes. Even young children can have cataracts. In children this may be due to poor glucose balance. However, most people do not develop cataracts until they are much older. A cataract is a collection of debris inside the lens of the eye. The lens of the eye resembles that of a camera. If your camera lens is dirty you cannot see through it and the same applies in the eye. Cataracts can cause blurred vision. Sometimes the blurring is patchy.

Your doctor will check your visual acuity by asking you to read letters off an eye chart – 6/6 or 6/5 is good and then look at your eyes in a darkened room, usually after putting drops in to dilate (widen) the pupil. The drops (usually tropicamide) will wear off gradually or can be reversed but do not drive until you can see normally. You should not be driving if your vision has deteriorated badly. Can you still fulfil visual requirements for the driving test? When the cataract is 'ripe' an eye surgeon (opthalmologist) will remove the lens under local or general anaesthetic. Often an artificial lens will be inserted in its place.

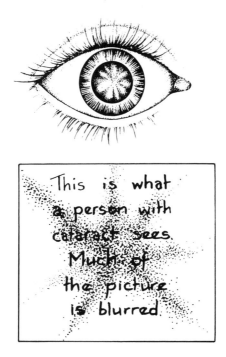

Cataracts

125

Diabetic retinopathy Retinopathy is one of the major complications of diabetes. It means disorders due to diabetes affecting the back of the eye. The retina is the part we see with (like the film in a camera). Diabetes is the most common cause of blindness in people of working age in Britain, but this situation is gradually improving. The development of diabetic retinopathy can be delayed or even avoided by keeping your blood glucose normal. And even if it does develop it can be treated successfully. After 15 years of diabetes virtually all insulin-treated diabetics will have some evidence of diabetic retinopathy. After 15 years of non-insulin requiring diabetes, about 65 per cent will have some evidence of retinopathy. However, in many people this will simply be tiny red dots which do not affect vision.

Eye checks People with diabetes must have their eyes checked at least once a year. They can be checked in several ways, but the essential is for someone to look at the retina either with a special torch called an ophthalmoscope and/or by taking a photograph. In most instances this has to be done in a dark room after eye drops have been put in to dilate your pupil. To use the ophthalmoscope the observer (who may be a doctor, optometrist, ophthalmic optician or specially trained nurse) must come close to you and look through the black pupil in the centre of your eye. He will ask you to look straight ahead, and it makes it much easier if you can fix on a point ahead and keep looking in that direction even if his head is in the way. You can blink, but do not forget to breathe! Another way of checking is to take a photograph of the eye with a camera which focuses on your retina using infra-red light. This is called non-mydriatic retinal photography because it is usually done without needing to put eye drops in.

Background retinopathy This is the commonest form of diabetic retinopathy. At first all that can be seen are swollen veins. As the condition progresses, microaneurysms (tiny red dots near blood vessels) and haemorrhages (red smudges or blots) are found, alone or with fatty yellow exudates. Background retinopathy does not usually cause any loss of vision – you are unlikely to know you have it. However, it can progress to more severe problems so must be detected and watched carefully. If the exudates are over the macula (the area of best vision) they can reduce vision (see below).

The treatment of background retinopathy is a gentle return of your blood glucose to normal. Once this has been achieved, then keep it there.

Macular disease The macula is a tiny area of retina where the best vision is concentrated. It can become swollen (macular oedema) or exudates can block the path of light or encircle it. If the macula is affected visual acuity will be reduced and you will notice a problem. An ophthalmologist (eye doctor) may be able to improve matters with laser treatment. Again, you must gently return your blood glucose to normal.

Pre-proliferative and proliferative retinopathy This is the most serious form of diabetic eye disease. Pre-proliferative retinopathy is shown by irregular veins and soft white blobs on the retina – soft exudates or cotton-wool spots. One in two people with these changes develop proliferative retinopathy in two years. In proliferative retinopathy new blood vessels grow across the retina or out forwards into the clear jelly or vitreous through which we see. These new vessels are fragile and bleed easily, filling the vitreous with blood through which you cannot see. The new vessels can also cause fibrous tissue which drags the retina off its supporting tissue – retinal detachment. Up to one in four people with new vessels will lose vision in that eye in the next two years. Urgent laser treatment – within weeks – can greatly reduce the risk of blindness from proliferative retinopathy.

Unfortunately you may have no symptoms of pre-proliferative retinopathy or proliferative retinopathy until it is too late. Once a bleed has occurred you will either see a black film across your vision or black floaters across it. If you see anything like this you must see your doctor that day or go to the emergency department of an eye

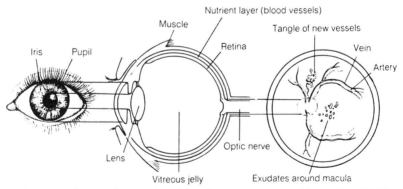

In the centre is a vertical section through a normal eye, while on the right is what the doctor sees when he looks through the pupil of someone with severe diabetic retinopathy

hospital. Urgent treatment may save your vision. If the retina is being pulled off its supports it may be possible to remove the vitreous and stop any further traction on the sensitive retina. This is called vitrectomy.

Laser treatment is usually done as an out-patient procedure, with some local anaesthetic in the eye. The dilating drops needed can blur your vision for a while. The laser treatment does not hurt but it may make your eye ache or give you a headache.

Other eye problems Clots in the arteries or veins in the retina are more common in people with diabetes than others, as is glaucoma. Glaucoma is an increase of pressure in the vitreous fluid bathing the inside of the eye. If you have a painful, tense, red eye you must go to your doctor immediately. Less dramatic signs of glaucoma are halos around lights, blurred vision and eye ache. Glaucoma is diagnosed by dropping local anaesthetic onto the eye and putting a measuring device called a tonometer onto the numbed cornea. It is readily treated.

WARNING
Doctors need to use eye drops to dilate (widen) the pupil of the eye to see the retina. This may be dangerous in people who have:

- Glaucoma;
- A previous eye operation;
- An artificial lens implanted during a cataract operation.

If you have any of these make sure you warn anyone about to put drops in your eyes – before they put the drops in!

Ears

Deafness Deafness is not always recognised as being linked with diabetes, but the auditory nerves can be damaged by diabetes and cause hearing impairment. A hearing test will determine the type of problem and, if necessary, a hearing aid can be fitted.

Neck

The back of the neck is a classical site for carbuncles or boils. At the front, the thyroid gland may swell, indicating possible thyroid overactivity.

CHEST

The chest contains the heart and lungs, confined within the ribs which are linked to the breastbone or sternum with springy cartilage. The underside of the chest cavity is formed by the muscular diaphragm. The oesophagus or gullet runs behind the heart and in front of the backbone or spine, carrying food from the mouth to the stomach.

Heart

Chest pain Most pains in the chest are not due to heart disease. The problem with describing symptoms in detail is that we all start feeling them as soon as we read about them – it is an occupational hazard for doctors and nurses. So don't start imagining things. Classically heart pain is a tight, crushing pain in the centre of the chest radiating across the chest and sometimes up the neck to the jaw or down the arms,

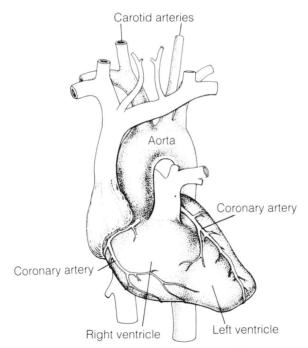

The heart, showing the major arteries leaving it and the coronary arteries which supply the heart itself

usually the left. Because diabetes can affect the nerves, heart pain may not be classical in diabetics.

Angina Angina means tightness or narrowness – thus angina pectoris is tightness of the chest. This is a sign that part of your heart is not getting enough blood. Symptoms can be chest tightness, radiating to the neck or arms, which occurs with exercise, agitation, excitement or emotion – anything which makes your heart pound. Angina can be relieved by glyceryl trinitrate tablets or spray under the tongue. Pills such as nitrates, beta blockers (e.g. atenolol) and calcium channel antagonists (e.g. nifedipine) may prevent angina attacks.

Heart attack This is a non-specific name for the acute condition in which a clot in an artery supplying part of the heart muscle (coronary thrombosis) causes the muscle that artery supplies to die (myocardial infarction). This causes the same sort of pain that occurs in angina, but often more severe and prolonged. Angina is a temporary condition. A myocardial infarct is permanent. Other symptoms of myocardial infarction are being very frightened, sweating, nausea or vomiting, burping and shortness of breath. Some people have minor symptoms only.

Nowadays, there is a specific treatment for coronary thrombosis – thrombolysis or 'clot busting' drugs, e.g. streptokinase. People with retinal new vessels should avoid thrombolysis in case they bleed (page 127). The sooner thrombolytic treatment is injected into a vein, the more likely it is to prevent myocardial infarction – permanent heart muscle damage. It works best within six hours of the onset of the symptoms. So telephone your doctor immediately if you have symptoms of a heart attack. Electrocardiograms (ECGs) will confirm the diagnosis, as will later blood tests for enzymes leaking out of damaged heart cells. You will be kept under observation on a coronary care unit for a day or so, and will usually be given aspirin and beta blocker drugs (unless you are sensitive to them). You will gradually get up and about and most people leave hospital in about a week. Most hospitals have a coronary rehabilitation programme. Many doctors will check how your heart responds to exercise with an exercise ECG, to see if you need further treatment.

Coronary angiography is a common further investigation of angina or myocardial infarction. Dye is injected into your coronary arteries through a fine tube threaded up a groin artery to the heart. This is done under local anaesthetic with X-ray screening. You may feel hot when the dye is injected and may have a bruise on your leg. This will

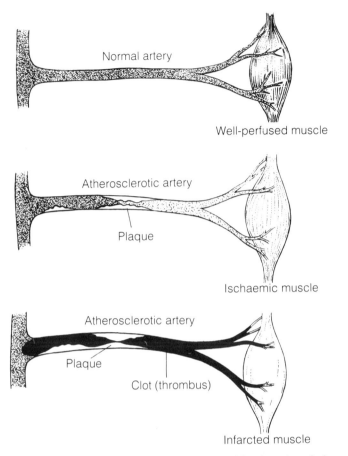

Normal artery

Well-perfused muscle

Atherosclerotic artery

Plaque

Ischaemic muscle

Atherosclerotic artery

Plaque

Clot (thrombus)

Infarcted muscle

Atherosclerosis. The artery becomes partly blocked by deposits of plaque on which clots may develop, blocking the artery completely. The muscle first becomes damaged and then dies completely

settle. If particular types of coronary artery narrowing are seen, angioplasty (stretching the narrowing with a balloon) or coronary artery bypass surgery may be recommended. Make sure you understand exactly what the cardiologist or cardiac surgeon plans to do and what any risks are.

Coronary thrombosis is a common condition from which the majority of people recover to continue working and enjoying their hobbies. It takes about two to three months to get back to normal and you should not drive for the first month, or until your doctor says you can. If you have angina or coronary thrombosis you must not smoke, must watch your weight and blood pressure and should eat a low fat diet. When your doctor agrees you should take regular exercise.

Lungs

Chest infection If you have a chest pain on one side of your chest or in the back of your chest, which hurts when you take a breath in, especially if you are coughing up green phlegm or are breathless, you may have an infection in your lung. Call your doctor. People with diabetes are prone to infection. Antibiotics will soon resolve it.

Breathlessness may simply be due to general lack of fitness or being overweight. It can be a sign of many chest problems, including asthma, bronchitis and infection. If you have sustained heart damage it can be due to water collecting in the lungs because the heart is not pumping vigorously enough to clear it. This is called pulmonary oedema or left ventricular failure and usually responds to diuretic pills. Diuretics make you pass urine and clear water (and sometimes potassium) from the body. They include frusemide and bumetanide.

ABDOMEN

This lies between the lower ribs and the groins and is commonly called the tummy or (inaccurately) the stomach. (See page 29). The real stomach lies inside the left abdominal cavity and delivers food to the duodenum and thence to the small intestine and the large intestine or colon. Faeces leave the body via the rectum. Behind the stomach lies the pancreas which drains its digestive juices into the duodenum. The liver lies under the ribs on the right. The gall bladder hangs below the liver from which it collects bile. The bile then drains into the duodenum to mix with the digestive enzymes from the pancreas. The kidneys are at the back of the abdominal cavity – one on each side. Urine drains from the kidneys down the ureters to the bladder which is at the bottom of the abdominal cavity, just inside the pubic bone. In a woman, the ovaries and uterus lie behind the bladder. The urine passes out through the urethra. The urethra is short in a woman and passes in front of the vagina, which is in front of the rectum. In men the urethra is longer because it travels through the penis. The testes hang in the scrotum to keep them cool. The blood supply for the abdominal

132

organs, and the legs, spurts down from the heart through the aorta which runs in front of the backbone. Used blood travels back up the vena cava – the great vein beside the aorta.

Gastrointestinal problems

Pancreatitis Pancreatitis is one cause of diabetes. It means inflammation of the pancreas and can cause very severe pain in the epigastrium – the part of the central abdomen just below the ribs. The pain may radiate to the back and be eased by sitting up. It is usually associated with vomiting. Chronic recurring pancreatitis may occur with several conditions including alcohol excess. Gall stones can cause pancreatitis too. A very high blood amylase level may support the diagnosis. Treatment is pain killers and fluid replacement through a vein.

Diabetic gastroparesis This means a partial paralysis of stomach emptying found in people with diabetes whose autonomic nerves are not working. The nerves are the cables which carry electronic signals to all parts of the body from the brain and which send messages back to the brain. The autonomic nerves are responsible for body functioning. If the stomach cannot empty you feel overfull after eating and may vomit often. This can be associated with indigestion pains. The treatment is good glucose balance and drugs such as metoclopramide or cisapride which encourage stomach emptying.

Diabetic diarrhoea This is another manifestation of autonomic neuropathy. It can wake you suddenly early in the morning and you may need to rush to the toilet several times. The treatment is good glucose balance and drugs like codeine which slow the bowel down. Antibiotics sometimes help.

Constipation Constipation can be due to dehydration, as in uncontrolled diabetes, or to failure of the nerves which tell the bowel muscles to move faeces along. Dehydration-induced constipation responds to fluid replacement. Laxatives or enemas can help the other kind.

Kidney and bladder problems

Infections Infections of the urinary tract and kidneys are more common in women than in men. This may be because a woman's short urethra can easily become contaminated with faecal organisms. However, diabetic men may also have urinary tract infections. Cystitis

133

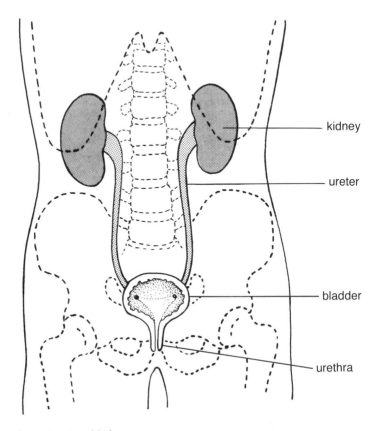

kidney

ureter

bladder

urethra

The urinary tract and kidneys

or bladder infection causes burning pain on passing urine, a sense of incomplete urination and the need to try to pass urine very frequently. The urine may be cloudy, or pink with blood, and smell horribly fishy.

Kidney infections or pyelonephritis may occur with or without symptoms of cystitis. You may have a high fever, vomiting and loin pain on the side of the affected kidney.

Antibiotics cure these infections. Cystitis rarely leads to hospital admission, but pyelonephritis can make you ill enough to warrant this. The blood glucose may rise and you may need more insulin or glucose-lowering tablets. You must drink plenty of clear fluids. Potassium citrate sometimes relieves the symptoms. If you have recurrent urinary tract infections be especially careful about perineal hygiene – women should wipe or wash from urethra to anus and not the other way round. Do not use strong soap in this sensitive area. Men should be careful to clean gently under the foreskin.

Nephropathy Nephropathy means kidney disease. The kidneys act as filters for water, salts and waste products. Blood is delivered in tiny tangles of blood vessels called glomeruli. Wastes, salt and water filter out of the blood vessels into collecting chambers and thence through concentrating tubules to the main drainage system to the kidneys. This urine then passes through the ureters to the bladder. In diabetes the walls of the blood vessels or capillaries thicken or become irregular. Wastes can no longer filter out to make urine. In other instances proteins leak out – in very small amounts to produce microalbuminuria, and then in larger amounts to produce frank proteinuria. Dipstick urine tests can detect this protein leak. If you are losing a lot of protein, your blood albumin level will fall and you will be unable to keep water inside the bloodstream. You will develop swelling of the ankles, legs, face and elsewhere. This is called nephrotic syndrome.

You have millions of glomeruli in each of two kidneys so it may be many years (if ever) before you notice any ill effects of diabetic

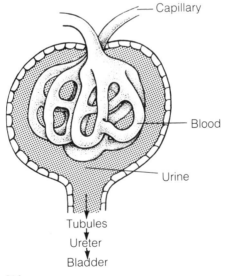

A glomerulus in the kidney

135

nephropathy. If the glomeruli are all damaged the wastes will build up in your blood. You may become tired and nauseated with itchy skin and a lack of energy. You may develop shortness of breath, either because of fluid build-up or because the accumulation of wastes makes your blood acid. In particular, blood urea and creatinine concentrations will rise, as may blood potassium level. Your doctor will ask you to save all your urine for 24 hours and have a simultaneous blood sample taken to calculate the kidney clearance of creatinine from the blood into the urine.

As all these changes occur, the kidney damage may cause your blood pressure to rise, which can cause further kidney damage. In order to stop this vicious circle it is vital to keep your blood pressure normal (see page 140).

There are many causes of kidney disease and your doctor will want to be sure that yours is due to diabetes and not a condition requiring different treatment. Diabetic nephropathy is virtually always linked with diabetic retinopathy (see page 126). You will probably have an ultrasound scan, and perhaps an intravenous urogram to check kidney size, drainage and function.

Treatment depends on exactly what your problem is. Is it mainly protein loss and hence fluid build-up? Or is it accumulation of wastes? Initially good control of blood glucose and blood pressure, a diet, correct fluid balance, instant treatment of urinary tract and other infections may be all that is needed to manage diabetic nephropathy. Diuretics can help in some cases. If the condition progresses you may eventually need peritoneal dialysis or haemodialysis. Renal transplant is successful in treating renal failure in people with diabetes.

Bladder problems Such problems may include urinary incontinence and difficulty in emptying the bladder. In someone who has difficulty preventing urine leaks, a high blood glucose can cause increased urine flow and, especially in children or elderly people, urinary incontinence. Leaks can also occur if bladder sensation is lost through diabetic nerve damage. Nerve damage, autonomic neuropathy, can make it difficult to squeeze all the urine out of the bladder. If this is a problem, try pressing down behind the pubic bone to complete bladder emptying.

SEXUAL PROBLEMS AND PERIODS

Libido

Sex drive or libido can be diminished in anyone who is ill (for example with uncontrolled diabetes) and usually returns as you recover. If this problem persists, your doctor can check your sex hormone levels.

Menstruation

Periods (menstruation) can become irregular or stop in someone with undiagnosed or uncontrolled diabetes. They usually return to normal as the diabetes comes under control. Periods and the menopause can affect glucose balance (see page 118).

Pregnancy

Pregnancy is not a complication of diabetes – but diabetes and pregnancy can complicate each other – see Chapter 16.

Impotence

Impotence has many causes, and can affect most men at some times in their lives. In many instances a temporary inability to achieve an erection is due to emotional factors or the circumstances in which you are trying to have intercourse. Patience and an under-standing partner can often resolve this sort of impotence. General ill-health, whether diabetes-related or not, can cause temporary impotence.

If you have no erections at all, whether with masturbation, spontaneously during the night, on waking, or when with a partner, it is more likely that you have a hormonal or mechanical sexual problem. If you are short of the male sex hormone, testosterone, this can be replaced to restore your sex life in most cases. Testosterone is useless in other cases – it increases the desire but not the performance. In diabetes, the problem may be inadequate blood supply to the penis due to furring up of the arteries, or to lack of the nerve signals which tell the penis to become erect. Arterial problems can sometimes be treated by vascular surgery. Occasionally, nerve problems improve with improved blood glucose balance. However, in some instances, the nerve damage is permanent.

There are many treatments for impotence. The simplest are double sheaths which allow a small vacuum to be induced (either by you sucking on an air tube, or by a pump). This vacuum draws blood into the penis which keeps it erect. These devices include Correcaid, Erecaid and Pos-T-Vac. Most manufacturers supply a made-to-measure device and aftersales advice. Another treatment is to inject papaverine into the base of the penis. This induces erection in about 20 minutes and the dose can be adjusted to suit you. Rarely, papaverine causes an unduly prolonged and painful erection. Some men find that as their confidence improves they can have erections without the papaverine. Some surgeons implant silicon tubes or other devices to stiffen the penis, but it would seem sensible to try non-invasive methods first.

Impotence is an emotive subject. Often men do not want to talk it over with their wives or partners, but it is nearly always best to be open with each other. And your wife may be greatly relieved to know that you do still love her but have avoided sex only because you have a physical problem. Some couples find renewed pleasure in non-penetrative sexual activities. Others enjoy non-sexual pastimes together.

It is also sensible to tell your doctor about your worries. He or she will not be embarrassed and can always help. Many hospitals have a counselling service. Some have impotence clinics.

Infections

Thrush This can cause perineal itching and burning in diabetic men and women and can be passed on during sexual contact. It can make your skin red and sore, and causes a creamy curd-like discharge. It is easily treated by antifungal creams which should be given to both partners for a full course of treatment. Women should ensure that the cream is also put into the vagina. The thrush fungus is common and seems to like a sugary, moist environment.

ARMS AND LEGS

Joints and tendons

Cheiroarthropathy This means stiff hand joints. It can also occur in the toes. It rarely limits what you can do. It is due to tightening of the ligaments in the fingers. The same process can cause claw toes. Try finger exercises in the warm to keep your fingers supple.

Dupuytren's contracture This is a similar process causing tightening of the tendons in the palm. It occurs in non-diabetics as an inherited problem and sometimes with other conditions.

Problems with nerves

Peripheral neuropathy Peripheral neuropathy is nerve damage occurring in the nerves supplying the extremities or periphery of the body. The whole body is served by nerves. Some carry instructions from the brain to the body. These are called motor nerves. Other nerves carry information to the brain from body and skin sensors. They are called sensory nerves. The autonomic nerves carry signals to the heart, blood vessels, gut, bladder, for example. In diabetes, sorbitol and other abnormal substances can be deposited inside the nerve. The nerve sheath can be damaged, and its blood supply may become erratic. All this impairs transmission of the electronic signals running up or down nerves. This may mean that no signals get through or that they are scrambled and send misleading messages to your brain.

Sensory neuropathy is the commonest form. It can affect any

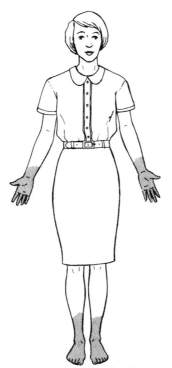

The extent of numbness in someone with glove and stocking peripheral neuropathy

sensory modality – touch, temperature, pain, vibration or position. The feet are more often affected than the hands. Classically people with diabetes develop a 'glove or stocking neuropathy'. You may feel tingling or pins and needles in your feet or hands. Occasionally this can be painful. You may develop numbness, sometimes so marked that you can injure your foot and not notice. You may not to able to tell if your bath is too hot. Some people do not know exactly where their feet are in relation to the ground – rather like walking on cotton-wool. Your doctor will test sensation with sterile pins, wisps of cotton wool or the vibration from a tuning fork. Absence of ankle reflexes may also indicate neuropathy.

Motor neuropathy is less frequent. It can affect one muscle or a group of muscles. If their nerve supply is interrupted they become atrophied and weak or paralysed. In diabetic amyotrophy, the thigh muscles are affected in this way.

There are many causes of neuropathy other than diabetes (including vitamins B_{12} deficiency and alcohol) so these must be excluded. Good glucose balance is essential and may relieve tingling. Many drugs have been tried. Antidepressants like amitriptylline are effective – not because you are depressed but because of a specific effect on the nerves and receptors. Other agents like carbamazepine can relieve neuralgic pain. If you have loss of sensation you must protect the numb area(s) from injury and inspect them regularly.

Carpal tunnel syndrome This describes the trapping of the median nerve as it runs through a fibrous tunnel at the wrist. This entrapment causes pain or tingling in the thumb and next one and a half fingers. Symptoms are often worse at night. It can also cause finger weakness. A simple operation can release the trapped nerve.

Circulatory problems

High blood pressure High blood pressure is included in this section because it is usually measured by a cuff around the upper arm (see page 21). Of course, your blood pressure exerts effects all around your circulation. You may be completely unaware that your blood pressure is high until it has exerted considerable damage on your heart and kidneys.

A doctor or nurse must check your blood pressure regularly – or you can buy a blood pressure machine (sphygmomanometer) and learn how to measure it yourself if you wish. High blood pressure – hypertension – is treated with beta blockers (best avoided in insulin-treated diabetics, see page 111), calcium channel antagonists (e.g. nifedipine), thiazide diuretics inappropriate for some diabetics because they raise the blood glucose) and ACE inhibitors (e.g. captoril, enalapril etc.) ACE inhibitors are thought to help protect your kidneys and are being used increasingly in diabetes. Keep your weight normal, do not smoke and eat a low salt, low fat diet.

Postural hypotension If you have autonomic nerve damage your blood pressure may fall when you stand up. This can cause dizziness or fainting.

Peripheral vascular disease This problem is not confined to diabetics. It also troubles smokers and people with high blood fats. If the arteries supplying the legs become atherosclerotic (furred up) blood flow to the legs and feet is reduced. This may cause pain in the calves on walking – intermittent claudication (intermittent limping). The pain comes on sooner going upstairs or uphill and is eased by rest. If the blood flow is severely restricted you may develop sluggish circulation in your feet – they become very white if you raise them and take a long time to regain their colour on lowering. Eventually they take on a reddish tinge and may start to hurt at night so that you have to hang them over the bedside. If you have this type of rest pain you must call your doctor urgently. If the circulation is completely blocked you will develop gangrene. Signs of this are bluish purple discoloration followed by blackening. Fortunately this is rare. As with rest pain, this is a medical emergency. Call your doctor now.

Stopping smoking is essential – indeed some vascular surgeons may not treat people who continue to smoke. A low fat diet is sensible. Continued exercise may encourage collateral vessels to develop and the intermittent claudication may improve. So keep walking if you can (don't forget to protect your feet). Your doctor will examine your pulses and may listen to them with an ultrasound probe resting lightly on the skin. X-rays recording the flow of dye injected into a groin artery under local anaesthetic may show a narrowing which can be relieved by stretching with a balloon (angioplasty) or by a bypass operation. If there is a clot it can sometimes be dissolved (see page 130). If you have developed gangrene it is virtually impossible to rescue that toe or foot and it will probably have to be amputated. Because your circulation is very poor a local amputation may not heal and your surgeon may advise a below knee amputation. However, advances in surgical techniques to improve the circulation may reduce the risk of major amputation. With good healing, expert rehabilitation

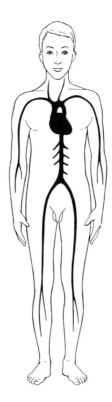

The major arteries

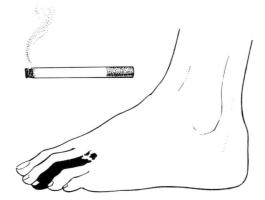

A gangrenous toe in a smoker with diabetes

142

advice and vigorous physiotherapy you can learn to walk (with an artificial limb if necessary) and could be expected to return to most jobs within a few months.

Diabetic foot problems

As can be seen from the descriptions above your feet are very vulnerable. These are some potential problems:

- Claw toes;
- Numbness;
- Insensitivity to temperature;
- Clumsiness because of poor position sense;
- Abnormal gait because of the above;
- Abnormal weight distribution causing rubbing or callus;
- Poor circulation;
- Poor healing.

These can lead to small rubs and wounds which you may not notice and which soon become infected. It is therefore vital that you learn to look after your feet.

Examine your feet every day. Sit comfortably. Take your shoes, socks or tights off and look at the top and bottom of your feet very carefully in a good light. Do not forget to look at the tips of each toe and in between the toes. If you cannot see your feet properly or cannot get close enough, ask someone to help you. Sometimes a mirror can help. Is the skin red? Is it broken anywhere? Are there blisters? Is there skin thickening on the sole or elsewhere? Is there any swelling? Do you have athletes' foot? Touch your feet – can you feel touch? Are they cold? Are there local areas of hotness?

Wash your feet every day in lukewarm water and dry them very carefully, especially between the toes. Cut your toenails regularly, being very careful to cut them straight across without sharp points or edges which could dig into the sides of that toe or other toes. Put on clean socks or tights each day. Socks should be made of wool or cotton. Never wear nylon socks – they can rub and they do not absorb sweat so the feet can get soggy. Ensure that your socks or tights are loose enough for all your toes to wriggle freely and that socks do not cause a tight ring around your ankle. (Ladies should never use garters to hold up stockings.) Buy shoes which feel comfortable in the shoe shop and that cannot rub you or pinch you anywhere. Very high heeled or pointed toe shoes are not suitable for diabetics. Do not wear

143

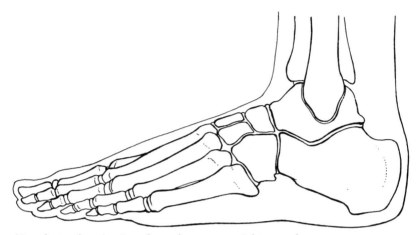

Your foot – these intricate bones bear your weight everyday

sandals – they increase the risk of small injuries. Use a shop which has a professional shoe fitter. If you work in the construction industry or sites or factories where there is a risk of foot injury wear comfortable professional protective footwear (e.g. steel toe-caps). Ask your chiropodist for advice. Never use a hot water bottle in bed – use an electric blanket with a thermostat and turn it off before you get in. Never get into a hot bath unless you have checked the temperature with a bath thermometer. You should see a chiropodist regularly – this means at least once a year and more often for those who cannot care for their own feet or who have 'at risk feet' – i.e. any of the problems listed above or who have ever had a foot ulcer or injury.

If you notice any change in your feet, discuss it with your chiropodist. Any breaks in the skin, however small, should be cleaned, covered by a non-adherent dressing (e.g. N-A) and checked daily. If injuries do not heal rapidly, start oozing pus or become surrounded by redness, you need to see a doctor straightaway because you probably need antibiotics. If in doubt contact your doctor. Wound care in diabetes requires expertise and experience. Some hospitals have wound care sisters or dressing clinics. Some chiropodists take a special interest in diabetes. Once the wound has been dressed, keep off it. This can mean resting for weeks, but if you walk on an ulcer it rarely heals. Total contact plaster casts can be used to redistribute the weight but must be applied only by experts. When you are resting your foot, put it up on a stool or sofa. Make sure that you do not rest the weight of your leg on your heel – you may get a pressure ulcer there. Support

144

your whole calf (e.g. with a plastic foam trough or wedge) and leave the heel free from the bed or stool.

In someone with diabetes a tiny foot ulcer can cause trouble out of all proportion to its size. It may lead to severe skin and tissue infection, bone infection (osteomyelitis), blood poisoning and amputation. Look after your feet well and seek early advice about all problems, however minor.

Charcot joints Charcot joints are a bone problem which can occur in anyone with severe lower limb neuropathy. People with neuropathy sometimes ignore minor injuries because they do not feel pain properly. The neuropathy alters the circulation within the bone and makes it weaker. Walking on a minor injury causes damage to the thin bones and fractures can develop. The joints may gradually be destroyed. The joint becomes red and swollen and may eventually become mis-shapen. If you have diabetic neuropathy in your feet and have persistent problems after a minor injury, or an unexpected injury to your feet or ankles, insist on an X-ray. The management of Charcot joints usually requires a combination of orthopaedic surgeon and diabetes team.

SUMMARY

- Diabetes is a multi-system disorder.
- It can affect all the major body systems.
- These effects include problems with skin, eyes, heart, kidneys, stomach, bowels, sexual functions, blood vessels, blood pressure, muscles, nerves and ligaments and joints.
- Feet and eyes are especially vulnerable.
- The longer you have had diabetes, the more likely you are to have diabetic tissue damage.
- Most people are NOT seriously troubled by tissue damage, but many require treatment for various aspects.
- Learn to check your body and report problems early.
- Attend your medical checks, even if you feel perfectly well.
- Diabetic tissue damage is not inevitable, you can greatly reduce the likelihood of being affected. The next chapter will tell you how.

13

PREVENTING DIABETIC TISSUE DAMAGE

We still have a lot to learn about diabetic tissue damage – thousands of people in many countries are researching in this area. However, some factors have been identified as being definitely or probably related to the development and progression of tissue damage in people with diabetes. You can do something about them. Do not wait until it is too late. All diabetic tissue damage becomes more likely with time. The longer you have had your diabetes, the more likely you are to have tissue damage. Virtually every person with diabetes will have some evidence of diabetic tissue damage eventually. What you do now will affect your health and well-being in years to come. The choice is yours.

STOP SMOKING

There is no doubt about the harmful effects of smoking. One in five of all deaths in the United Kingdom is due to cigarette smoking. Of 1000 young men who smoke, approximately six will die on the roads, one will be murdered, and 250 will be killed by their cigarettes. Women are catching up fast. So, cigarettes kill one in four of those who smoke. Cigarettes also maim people. They cause cancers, for example in the lung, from which many people die a painful and lingering death. They fur up your arteries causing strokes, intermittent claudication (pain in the legs on walking), gangrene and amputation.

But if you have diabetes the risk is even greater. Your diabetes increases the likelihood of atherosclerosis causing coronary thrombosis and circulatory problems. If you smoke as well your risks of dying

146

from a coronary thrombosis are enormously increased. In addition to increasing your risk of death or disability, cigarettes can upset your blood glucose balance because the nicotine and other substances cause acute circulatory effects. For example, smoking a cigarette may upset your insulin absorption. Smoking can increase your blood fats. And smoking also poisons anyone who breathes in your smoke: if your wife does not smoke she is more likely to die of lung cancer than if she had married a non-smoker. The same applies to your children.

If you retain only one piece of advice from this book it should be this: DIABETICS DO NOT SMOKE. If you smoke, stop now, as you read this. And you will improve both your health and that of those around you.

LOSE WEIGHT

Take all your clothes off and stand in front of your mirror. Be completely honest with yourself. Are you fat? If you are then your fatness is not only increasing your risk of having a coronary thrombosis or high blood pressure, but also it makes your diabetes harder to control. Seek your dietitian's help in losing weight. Once you have reached the right weight for your height, stay there.

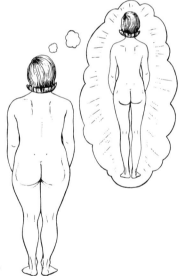

Be honest with yourself

147

KEEP YOUR BLOOD GLUCOSE CONCENTRATION NORMAL

People with high blood glucose levels are much more likely to develop diabetic retinopathy, diabetic nephropathy and diabetic neuropathy than those with normal blood glucose levels. The higher the glucose, and the longer it is high, the more likely you are to have one of these forms of tissue damage. If you have been running blood glucose levels persistently over 8 mmol/l (144 mg/dl) gradually reduce your blood glucose by decreasing your diet (if you are overweight), increasing your exercise and increasing your dose of insulin or glucose-lowering pills. See Chapters 8 and 9, and ask your diabetes adviser for help. Do not reduce your blood glucose abruptly – ease it down gradually over a few weeks. Two studies – the Diabetes Control and Complications Trial and the UK Prospective Diabetes Study are currently investigating the effects of glucose control on long-term tissue damage.

LOWER YOUR BLOOD FATS

Another word for blood fats is lipids. Your blood fats are cholesterol (mostly made up of the 'good' high density lipoprotein cholesterol or HDL, and the 'bad' low density lipoprotein cholesterol LDL) and triglyceride. If your total cholesterol is high with a low HDL and a high LDL; or if your triglyceride is high (especially in the presence of a low HDL), you are at risk of having a coronary thrombosis. The risk increases as the levels move away from the desirable range. This range will vary a little from laboratory to laboratory.

> Total cholesterol 3.5–5.2 mmol/l (135–200 mg/dl)
> HDL cholesterol > 0.9 mmol/l (35 mg/dl)
> LDL cholesterol < 5.0 mmol/l (193 mg/dl)
>
> Triglyceride < 2.3 mmol/l (203 mg/dl)

If your total cholesterol is over 7.8 mmol/l (300 mg/dl) you are at very high risk of having a coronary thrombosis. You can improve your blood fat levels by keeping your weight normal, and by eating much less fat. The fat that you do eat should be high in polyunsaturates (e.g. sunflower oil) and monosaturates (e.g. olive oil), and low in saturated fat (animal and dairy fat, see page 62). A high fibre diet helps too. Reducing your sugar and alcohol intake helps to reduce your triglyceride level. Exercise will help too, and *you must stop smoking*.

KEEP YOUR BLOOD PRESSURE NORMAL

High blood pressure increases the likelihood of developing athero-sclerosis. Coronary thromboses and strokes are commoner in people with hypertension than in those whose blood pressure is low. Keeping your weight normal and exercising regularly will help to keep your blood pressure down, and you should not add extra salt to your food at table or eat a lot of very salty food. It is important to have your blood pressure measured at least once a year. If it is persistently over 140/90 your doctor will consider blood pressure-lowering pills. In non-diabetics, some doctors would not initiate treatment unless the blood pressure was over 140/100, but the risks of hypertension are greater for diabetics than for non-diabetics, and many diabetologists would start pill treatment for a diastolic blood pressure persistently above 90 in a young person.

EXERCISE REGULARLY

Regular, vigorous exercise helps to reduce the likelihood of having a coronary thrombosis. It also improves sensitivity to insulin, helps you to lose weight and helps to reduce your blood fats (see pages 62 and 179). Never start an exercise programme without first consulting your doctor. You should exercise at least three times a week to help significantly.

NOTICE WHAT IS HAPPENING TO YOU – AND ACT

Darren was a bricklayer. He led a busy life. At work all day, out every evening with his girlfriend. He injected his insulin twice a day and did the occasional blood test. They were usually high but he felt OK. One day while he was changing to go out he felt something wet on his sock. It was blood. When he looked at his foot his big toe was all red and there was a hole underneath, with pus and blood coming out of it. He washed it and covered it with elastoplast, finished dressing and rushed out to the party. His toe did not seem to hurt much, and it did not stop him dancing. Two days later he started to feel ill. He felt hot and sweaty and shivery. His glucose was over 22 mmol/l (396 mg/dl). His mother called the doctor. When the doctor looked at his foot, it was red up to the ankle and there was pus oozing out of the toe. Darren spent the next six weeks in hospital. He had to have an operation to drain the pus and intravenous drips with antibiotics, and insulin. After he got home he looked at his working boots and found a nail sticking up through the insole. His toes had become numb from neuropathy and he had not noticed the nail digging in.

If Darren had checked his feet daily, he would have seen the early signs of injury in time to act. Had he taken more care of his blood glucose he may not have developed neuropathy.

This sort of story, sadly, is not uncommon. Every day diabetics are being admitted to hospitals in Britain with problems due to self-neglect. No one expects you to do everything perfectly – and there will be days when you forget things. But try to develop a routine for checking your body over and learn to notice what your skin looks like and what you feel like. If something is wrong you will often be able to sort it out yourself, but the diabetes team are always there to help – and they like to be asked. The aim is not to turn you into a hypochondriac, but to have an observant, common sense approach to what is going on in your body. If you discover a problem, he prepared to admit to yourself and your advisers that all is not well, then seek help if needed and act on it.

SUMMARY

- Keep fit. Prevent diabetic tissue damage.
- If you smoke, STOP. If you don't smoke, don't start.
- Keep your weight normal.
- Keep your blood glucose concentration normal.
- Keep your blood fats satisfactory.
- Keep your blood pressure normal.
- Keep exercising.
- Keep an eye on yourself.
- Be realistic.
- Be kind to yourself.

14

LIVING WITH DIABETES

A DAILY ROUTINE

Once you have got over the surprise of having discovered that you have diabetes and have learned the basics of looking after yourself you need to get back to enjoying life. But you must give your diabetes a little attention each day.

Establish a daily routine. Keep all your diabetes things together in a box, case or bag. Insulin-treated people should keep their spare insulin in a small box in the fridge (away from the freezing compartment).

A diabetes kit

At home your diabetes kit should include:

- Your diabetes record book and a pen;
- Your insulin, pen or syringe and needles;
- Alcohol swabs (or industrial methylated spirit) to clean insulin bottle bung;
- A needle clipper (B-D Safe Clip);
- Your pills;
- Your finger pricker, platforms (if needed) and lancets;
- Your blood glucose test strips, bottle, meter or biosensor;
- Cotton wool (if needed);
- A container for sharps;
- Urine testing kit for ketones (and glucose);
- A sparse diabetic card;
- Your help telephone numbers;
- Some spare glucose tablets;
- Your glucagon while you are at home.

Keep your diabetes kit out of reach of children – lock it away if there are children in your house. If the person with diabetes is a child, make sure his/her brothers and sisters cannot access the items. It is always sensible to have two of everything in case of breakages or loss (keep your reserve items in a separate place). If you are using an insulin-injection device, keep a syringe and needle in case of problems. You can draw insulin out of a cartridge if you have to.

Around town your diabetes kit should include:

- Your diabetes record book and pen;
- Insulin kit or that day's pills;
- Blood testing kit;
- Diabetic card;
- Glucose tablets;
- Your help telephone numbers;
- A fibre crunch bar or biscuits.

If you are often out and about you will probably find an insulin pen and a blood glucose biosensor easier to carry around than bottles of insulin, needles, syringes and a bottle of strips. See Chapter 18 for guidance on extended trips.

Tests and treatment

When you know what tests and treatment you need and when, decide how best to fit it into your daily routine. Most people test their blood (or urine) at least once a day, usually before a meal or before bed, sometimes two hours after the largest meal of the day. At first allow 5 to 10 minutes for each test and treatment time – you may soon be able to do blood tests in less than one minute and an insulin injection can take only a minute with a pen. Obviously people on diet alone or who take pills are at an advantage here. Now and then, it is worth spending a little time thinking whether you could make your testing and treatment easier for yourself or more efficient in any way. Where do you keep your diabetes things? Are they easy to reach and can you find what you want simply? Would another method of insulin injection suit you better? Are there problems with glucose testing? It is often the small things which can make a task a prolonged nuisance or a quick job.

Body maintenance

Choose a convenient time each day (e.g. before bed, or after your shower) to look at your feet carefully. Any time learn to listen to what the rest of your body is telling you – notice if you have problems seeing or feeling, notice if you have bowel or bladder problems and so on. But notice in a commonsense way. You do not need to become a hypochondriac:

'Do not distress yourself with imaginings. Many fears are born of fatigue and loneliness. Beyond a wholesome discipline, be gentle with yourself.'

Desiderata, 1692

Medical checks

From the outset you must accept that you will need to have routine checks with health care professionals. It is important to attend these sessions. Take time off work if necessary – your diabetes clinic will give you a letter if you need one for work. If you cannot attend, make certain you are given another date within a few weeks.

At least once a year:

- See a diabetes doctor;
- See a diabetes specialist nurse;
- See a dietitian;
- See an optometrist or ophthalmic optician;
- See a chiropodist.

You may need to see some of these people more often at some points in your diabetic career.

Arthur was a self-employed decorator. He worked hard. He became diabetic seven years ago and was treated with a diabetic diet and glibenclamide tablets. He last attended the diabetic clinic four years ago. He was too busy to waste time sitting around in clinic. 'Time is money,' he told his wife. He obtained his pills on repeat prescriptions and was always 'in a hurry – can't stop now, doc' when his GP suggested a check-up. Eventually the GP insisted. He was worried to discover that Arthur had diabetic retinopathy in both eyes. He asked him to have some blood taken and arranged a hospital visit. Arthur put the hospital appointment letter behind the clock and forgot it. He was sent another appointment – to no avail. His GP was told of his non-attendance and the hospital notes were returned to file.

One afternoon, Arthur arrived at the hospital in an ambulance. He had fallen off his ladder, knocked himself out and broken his leg in three places. When the casualty doctor tried to look in his eyes she couldn't see into the left one – it was full of blood. His blood glucose was 17 mmol/l (306 mg/dl) and his glycosylated haemoglobin was very high at 16 per cent. After Arthur regained consciousness he told staff what had happened. He had been unsteady on ladders for some time because 'my feet don't seem to feel where they are'. He had been painting the side of a house when he suddenly lost the vision in his left eye and as rapidly lost his balance. The vitreous haemorrhage (page 127) cleared and Arthur's fractures healed but he could no longer manage ladders and had to stop work.

Arthur's eye problems were treatable, he need never have had the haemorrhage into his eye. Had he followed his GP's advice and attended the clinic, he would probably still be working.

WORK

Applying for jobs

People with diabetes can do most jobs. Unless you have diabetic tissue damage (e.g. visual impairment or amputation) diet-treated diabetes should not affect your employment. People with diabetes treated with glucose-lowering pills or insulin injections cannot join the police, the armed forces or the fire service, or fly aircraft. Pill-treated diabetics may be allowed to drive trains, large goods vehicle (LGV) and passenger carrying vehicles (PCV) if you can show that you are caring for your diabetes properly, your glucose is well-balanced and you have no disabling tissue damage. If you are a vocational driver it is better to control your diabetes with metformin (page 76) if possible. Insulin-treated diabetics are not usually allowed to hold LGV or PCV licenses, drive trains, fly aircraft, become merchant sailors or divers. The risk, albeit small, of hypoglycaemia may also prevent your working at heights (e.g. circus acts, steeplejacks) or in jobs in which a lapse of attention could be dangerous, either for your own safety or that of others (e.g. working with hazardous machinery, or as a lighthouse keeper or signalman).

Diabetes is a registrable disability for employment but it may not be to your advantage to register – discuss this with your diabetes team, social worker or the British Diabetic Association.

Existing jobs

In most cases, no-one at work will realise that you now have diabetes, unless you tell them. If you are on glucose-lowering pills or insulin injections it is sensible to tell people with whom you spend a lot of time at work. In the unlikely event of your having a hypoglycaemic attack at work, they would then know what to do. If you are responsible for other people's safety and your diabetes is treated with insulin or sulphonylurea pills you *must* tell them about your diabetes. It is also sensible to tell your employer, so that you can have any time off that you need for medical reasons, and so that you can keep to your diet at work without difficulty.

Brian is a lively 20 year-old. He rarely had problems with his diabetes and saw no need to mention it at work. One morning he woke up late and missed his breakfast. He had his insulin and decided to have a snack at the travel agents where he works. There was a rush of customers and he forgot. Rita, his manageress, found him staggering around the office, sweating profusely and mumbling. He was trying to say 'sugar, give me sugar' but she did not understand. She panicked. Eventually a customer called an ambulance. The ambulance men found Brian's diabetic card and soon revived him with some glucose tablets.

Brian awoke to discover Rita in tears, 'I thought you were dying,' she sobbed. 'It was only a hypo, Rita' he said as he comforted her. When Rita had calmed down he told her about diabetes and hypos. He took her out to lunch to apologise.

If you are a vocational driver you must tell your employer, and the motor insurance company that you have diabetes. If you are already working in other jobs normally barred to diabetics you have a moral obligation, and often a contractual one, to report your diabetes to your employer. In many instances employers will be helpful and will allow you to continue in the job, perhaps in a safer role. You can also appeal against dismissal made on medical grounds – and such appeals can be successful. It is up to you to demonstrate that your diabetes is safely under control and that you can look after it responsibly. The British Diabetic Association can often help with employment-related matters.

Some people run into problems with company pension schemes or life insurance. There is a huge variation in the attitude of different insurance companies to people with diabetes. If you have problems the British Diabetic Association can usually help.

Studies of the work record of people with diabetes have produced varying results – one study in the early 1960s showed that about one in two men and one in three women with diabetes had no sick leave at all in a year. Another study showed that people with diabetes took less sick leave than the non-diabetics in their company. Employers are sometimes ignorant about diabetes – in the vast majority of cases they need have no worries about employing a person who has diabetes.

More detailed information for employees and employers can be found in *Fitness to Work – The Medical Aspects.* Edited by F.C. Edwards, R.I. McCallum and P.J. Taylor (A joint report of the Royal College of Physicians and the Faculty of Occupational Medicine, published by Oxford Medical Publications in 1988). The BDA also provides useful information.

Circumstances at work

There may be small changes which you can make to improve your circumstances at work. If the canteen food does not correspond to a healthy diabetic diet, take your own meals. Keep some emergency rations – biscuits, fibre-crunch bars, for example, in your desk or work box, if food is permitted in your workplace. Find somewhere clean to check your blood glucose or give your insulin. If your work involves uneven ground or heavy goods, consider protective footwear. If you have poor circulation, make sure that your feet are warm – there are regulations about the temperature of workplaces. If you are a non-smoker (and all diabetics should be) ask people not to smoke in your working area.

Shift work

There is no problem with this for solely diet-treated diabetics. If you are taking glucose-lowering pills, take them with your meals. It may be more difficult for persons with insulin-treated diabetes to work shifts, so try to avoid these if you can. However, if you do work shifts you can adjust your treatment to cover this. Most people find it easiest to take a very long-acting insulin once a day and use an insulin pen with fast-acting insulin before each meal. Then it is not so critical when you eat your meals. It is sensible to have snacks in between and to use frequent blood-glucose monitoring.

OTHER ASPECTS OF DAILY LIFE

Driving

This has already been discussed on pages 44 and 155. You must be especially careful not to endanger your life or that of others by driving when your blood glucose is too low, or by driving when you can no longer see properly, cannot feel the pedals or steering wheel, or when you have other diabetic tissue damage which interferes with driving. It is selfish (and illegal) to continue to drive when you are no longer a safe driver.

If you are on glucose-lowering pills or insulin, never drive on an empty stomach and, after any change in treatment, check your blood glucose before driving, and at hourly intervals during long journeys. Always carry glucose, food and a can or box of non-alcoholic drink in the car.

The instant you suspect you are hypoglycaemic, pull into the kerb or hard shoulder *immediately* it is safe to do so, turn off the engine and remove the keys from the ignition. Eat some glucose. Turn on the hazard warning lights. Slide into the passenger seat if you can. Eat some food. Do not resume your journey until your blood glucose is at least 6 mmol/l (108 mg/dl) and you are fully in control of yourself. If you are involved in an accident whilst hypoglycaemic you could be charged with driving whilst under the influence of a drug.

The old advice was for a hypoglycaemic person to get out of the car so that you are no longer 'in control' of it. However, with today's busy traffic, it is dangerous to advise someone who may be confused or inco-ordinated to leave the relative safety of their car and stagger into the traffic!

Social life

Eating out need not be a problem for people with diabetes. You can avoid sugary puddings by having fruit, and it is usually possible to choose a relatively low-fat meal – you do not have to eat the cream sauce! Most places will grill fish or steak, or provide a salad. And nowadays, most restaurants or hotels serve some wholemeal bread, muesli and other high fibre options. If you are invited out for a meal, politely explain beforehand to your host or hostess that you cannot eat very sugary or very fatty food. There are so many religious, personal and medical food preferences nowadays, that a wise hostess ask guests if they have any specific dietary requirements. Diabetes is no barrier to an active social life. Nowadays, there is no need to drink a

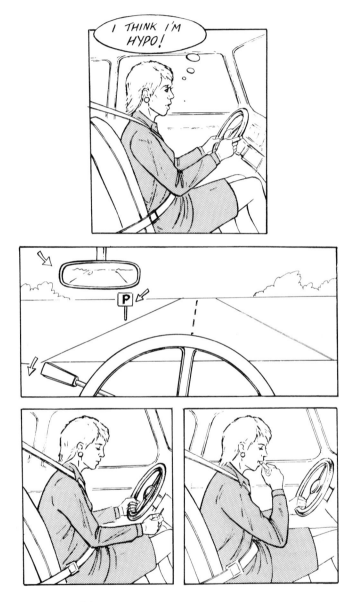

Hypoglycaemia and driving

lot of alcohol to be sociable. Space out your alcoholic drinks with non-alcoholic ones, and always have something to eat when you drink alcohol because alcohol inhibits the release of glucose from the liver and you could become hypoglycaemic.

Teenagers with diabetes can become angry and frustrated if their parents insist that they are home for meals and at injection times. If you make sure that you carry something to eat and if you use an insulin pen you do not need to rush home for meals and insulin and your social life can become a lot freer. Keep up to date with practical advances in diabetes care – they can make life much easier. This is one of many good reasons for joining your local diabetic association such as the BDA.

People are sometimes shy about discussing their diabetes with friends. Most people will be genuinely interested in your diabetes and how you look after it, if you wish to tell them. But remember that your friends may be shy of broaching the topic with you because they will not be sure whether you want to discuss it or not. Having diabetes does not stop you enjoying the same social life you have always had.

LIVING WITH DIABETES

During this century there have been many attitudes to diabetes by professionals and those who have it. Before the 1920s juvenile-onset diabetes was a death sentence. Once insulin was discovered there was a mood of great optimism – diabetes was no longer a problem. Joslin, a famous diabetes doctor, voiced a word of caution and predicted that diabetic tissue damage would gradually become more important. For people on insulin, early methods of treatment were painful and cumbersome – glass syringes and thick needles, complex methods of calculating the insulin dose, reliance on urine testing with all its inaccuracies. Then, with standardisation of insulin concentrations, easy self-monitoring of blood glucose and the advent of insulin pens, people with diabetes were again told that diabetes was no longer a problem, that they could do anything. People with diabetes who found the restrictions of insulin injections, self-testing and regular check-ups frustrating, or who could not achieve the smooth blood glucose balance promised by books and professionals, were made to feel as if they had failed in some way. They felt that it was wrong not to see life with diabetes through rose-tinted spectacles.

When glucose-lowering pills were discovered in the 1950s people whose diabetes could be controlled on these, and those requiring diet alone, were given the impression that their diabetes was only mild and not likely to cause them trouble. I had angry letters from people on pills when I wrote an article which said that there is no such thing as mild diabetes. Many of these people still have difficulty accepting that their foot or eye problems are due to diabetes. Others feel cheated – if it is a mild condition why are they in difficulties now? Now, many people with non-insulin-requiring diabetes want to have the same access to blood glucose monitoring and health care that insulin-treated people have, but there may still be resistance to this within the health care professions, especially in a budget-conscious world.

Nowadays, a balance is being struck between the reality of the need to give up some time and effort to looking after diabetes, the risk of tissue damage, and the possibility, in the majority of cases, of getting on with doing what you want in life and enjoying yourself to the full. There have been at least five diabetic presidents, innumerable diabetic sportsmen, company directors, singers, artists, musicians, builders, professors, doctors, nurses – the list is endless.

When I started writing books for people with diabetes it was not considered 'kind' to talk about tissue damage in detail. But to fail to do so seems to me to insult my readers' intelligence and to take away your opportunity to work towards reducing your risk of your diabetes causing long-term problems. The down side of giving such detailed information is that it provokes anxiety. A small trace of anxiety is what keeps one following health rules – I like eating, but I am stopped from stuffing myself every day by anxiety that I will get very fat and that will make me look horrible and I might die from a heart attack. I am not so anxious that I starve myself – it just keeps a small rein on my appetite. On the other hand, because my grandfather smoked and died of lung cancer I am so afraid that I might get cancer that I have never smoked. That is useful anxiety.

But too much worry and anxiety can be destructive.

Delia is 30 and has had diabetes for 15 years. She has always been a worrier, but in recent years she has been so frightened that she is going to develop kidney failure that she has been measuring her blood glucose six or more times a day and is always changing her insulin dose and omitting meals to lower her glucose. She is often severely hypoglycaemic because she tries to keep her glucose at 4 mmol/l (72 mg/dl) all the time. She had a car accident when she was hypoglycaemic and lost her driving licence. This meant that she became trapped in the village in which she lives as public transport is poor. Gradually she stopped going out. She missed some of her diabetic clinic appointments and the diabetic sister came out to her house to see how she was. Delia at first denied that there was a problem but eventually told the diabetic sister all her worries. She agreed to come to clinic where careful tests proved that her kidneys were working well. She was offered some sessions with a psychologist. She was terrified – 'you all think I'm mad,' she wept. But once she understood that these sessions were simply to help her to come to understand a little more about herself and her diabetes she agreed. The diabetes team helped her to reduce her hypoglycaemia by regular meals and appropriate insulin changes. She saw the psychologist regularly. Now, four years later, her blood glucose levels are normal much of the time, she has regained her driving licence and is working part-time. She still worries sometimes, but is able to cope with this and no longer allows anxiety to overcome her.

Norman is 20 and has also had diabetes for 15 years. His aunt was diabetic on insulin. He used to be taken to visit her when he was little. She was blind and walked with a white stick. She always walked with a limp and one day he fell against her leg and discovered that it was artificial. Despite all that the diabetes team taught him about the preventibilty of diabetic tissue damage, his childhood impressions were so strong that he always equated diabetes with inevitable blindness and amputation. He decided that if this was the future he would rather not know. He would have a short life and a merry one. He stopped attending diabetic clinic, never tested his blood glucose and gave himself some insulin once a day or so. As a result he had several episodes of ketoacidosis. During one of them he nearly died. He usually discharges himself from hospital as soon as he feels well enough to walk. On one occasion he ran out of the building when he was told that he needed to see the eye clinic urgently to treat his retinopathy. He rejected all offers of help. He moved house and was lost to follow-up. The diabetes team felt that they had failed because they had been unable to help him. On this occasion the psychologist working with the team helped the staff to accept that they could not help everyone. They needed to learn not to be too hard on themselves.

Every large diabetic clinic has two or three Delias and a few Normans (so I have combined their stories to protect individuals). Most people with diabetes are not so dramatically affected by their feelings. I have told these stories to show that feelings about diabetes can overwhelm a few people. Help is available. Not everyone needs a psychologist, and not every diabetes team is lucky enough to work with one. The first step is to find someone who understands about diabetes to share your worries with. If your worries have become so enormous that they have swamped you, professional help can rescue you so do not be afraid to admit to yourself and the diabetes team that you could do with help. We all do from time to time. We are all human and none of us is perfect.

Two Canadians, Heather Maclean and Barbara Oram, collected people's comments about their diabetes and discussed them in a book called *Living with Diabetes*. Not everyone they asked about diabetes viewed it as negative experience.

Lydia: 'I have a sense of having come to peace with my diabetes. I feel some sort of contentment. I think that has added to my sense of self-confidence. I feel now that I can do anything that I wish to put my hands on. There's a contentment about not having to think about diabetes any more, because it's a part of my life.'

Tim: 'I can say that diabetes has made me a better person. It's weird. I almost feel like I contradict myself when I say that because I hate diabetes, yet diabetes has made me a stronger person ... Since I got my diabetes things have really picked up for me. Diabetes has done so many things to me. I used to be on the shy side and now I'm not. I feel more confident in myself. It has strengthened me.'

Sarah: 'I know I'm better organized as a result of my diabetes, because I have to be – not only better organized to deal with diabetes but all around. There're certain things I have to do and that spills over into the rest of my life. I tend to think ahead a lot more than a lot of people, because I can't get caught in situations I can't handle. In a way, when I look at my life, there's positive things that balance out – like the organization, the diet – you have an extra incentive to eat well; also tuning into your own body. So I don't see it all as negative ... If I were given a chance to change one thing in my life and only one thing I can tell you right now that I wouldn't waste that chance on diabetes. I've never said that before but, in saying it now, I know absolutely that it's true.'

SUMMARY

- Establish a daily routine for your diabetes care.
- Keep your diabetes kit well-organised and safe.
- Make life easier for yourself – tailor your treatment and your monitoring to your personal needs.
- Take advantage of new advances.
- Have regular medical checks.
- People with diabetes can do most jobs.
- Tell close colleagues that you have diabetes.
- Tell your employer if the diabetes may affect your safety or that of others. It is best to tell employers anyway.
- Tell the DVLA that you have diabetes. Avoid hypoglycaemia while driving.
- Don't hide your feelings about your diabetes. Share them with people who understand. Accept help if you need it.
- Diabetes has some positive aspects.

15

THE DIABETES TEAM AND THE DIABETES SERVICE

Every clinic, surgery or health care service has a system. Learning how your particular care system actually works can help you to make full use of the facilities which may help you. It can also help you to understand why things happen as they do, and enable you to make suggestions for improvements if necessary.

Diabetes is a common condition which requires long-term care. This means that a hospital diabetic service can care for 1000 to 4000 patients depending on its catchment area and the availability of other clinics. A GP may have 10 to 100 diabetic patients, depending on his list type and size and whether he also cares for his partners' diabetic patients, for example. The potential size of diabetic clinics means that they have to be well-organised and that many staff are involved.

THE DIABETES TEAM

Nowadays, people with diabetes are cared for by a team of people, all of whom have particular skills. Different diabetes services have different teams, but most include a doctor with specialist training in diabetes, a diabetes specialist nurse, a dietitian, and a chiropodist. Some larger teams include people with skills in psychology, eye care and wound care, among others. Some team members may spend their whole time working with people with diabetes, others have additional responsibilities.

The most important team member

The most important team member is YOU. The traditional view of health care is that you, the patient, seek help from your doctor, who tells you what is wrong with you, and gives you treatment. 'I have a sore throat, doctor.' 'You have tonsillitis. Take one of these tablets four times a day for a week.' This approach is effective and perhaps sufficient in many conditions. But diabetes is a condition in which you, the person who has it, have a major influence on your own outcome. By eating healthily, exercising regularly, checking your condition regularly and adjusting your treatment according to your blood glucose levels, you can keep yourself well. You live with your diabetes all the time, so *you* can be the most knowledgeable person in the world about *your* diabetes. You are the most important member of the team.

Doctors

Nowadays, in Britain, no doctor aspiring to a hospital consultant post can be accredited in diabetes without stringent training. This occurs in hospital and usually includes one to three years training in various aspects of general medicine as a senior house officer, several years as a registrar in general medicine, including diabetes care and several years as a senior registrar in diabetes. Posts have to be approved by the Royal College of Physicians for higher medical training and must include broad general medicine and all aspects of diabetes care, both in-patients and out-patients. A period must be spent in research. As a consultant this doctor will then be a physician (everyone trained in general medicine is a physician and called 'Doctor' not 'Mister') with a special interest in diabetes, sometimes known as a diabetologist. Most diabetologists also practice general medicine. Those pursuing a career in academic medicine follow a similar pathway to start with but do more research. Some teaching hospitals have diabetologists at lecturer, senior lecturer or professorial level.

Not all hospitals have a consultant post specialising in diabetes. All general physicians will have some experience in diabetes care and sometimes the diabetic clinic is run by a general physician.

General practitioners undergo a broad training in several specialties at senior house officer level and then join a practice as a trainee, moving on to full partnership in a practice. Some GPs move into practice from registrar posts in medicine, some from specialised diabetes posts. Some work in hospital diabetic clinics as clinical assistants to a consultant diabetologist. There are courses in diabetes care for hospital doctors and GPs. There are also professional organisations (e.g. the medical and scientific section or the education section of the British Diabetic Association, the International Diabetes Federation) which offer excellent opportunities for updating knowledge, and for revision and peer review.

I believe that everyone with diabetes has the right to see a doctor specialising in diabetes care.

Nurses

One of the greatest advances in diabetes care has been the increase in the number of posts for nurses with specialist training in diabetes care. There are now over 500 such posts in Britain. A diabetes specialist nurse (or sometimes a diabetes specialist health visitor) has usually attended courses in diabetes care and spends all of her time caring for people with diabetes. She will often have received special training in teaching and is usually your main source of diabetes education. She will also know about all the practicalities of blood glucose testing, insulin administration and be able to advise you about adjusting your treatment. Diabetes specialist nurses usually work closely with a consultant diabetologist. Many diabetes specialist nurses will see you on the ward in hospital, in the clinic, at your GP's or at your home. They may give you an emergency number on which you can contact them for advice.

Nowadays it is becoming increasingly unusual to admit people to hospital to start insulin therapy. The diabetes specialist nurse can visit you at home and help you to learn how to manage your insulin.

Some practice nurses attend training courses in diabetes care and help with GP diabetic clinics. Community-based nurses such as district nurses may also have some diabetes training.

Dietician

Healthy eating is the cornerstone of the treatment of diabetes. Dieticians have detailed training in nutrition and its effects on the body. They will be able to assess your usual eating pattern and help you to adapt it to a diabetic diet. The dietician will not only advise you about the types of food to eat but also guide you about how best to cook them. If you have concerns about food safety or storage she can help there too.

Chiropodist

A chiropodist has received training in keeping your feet healthy and in assessing and treating any problems which arise. He may measure the sensation in your feet and check your circulation. He will be able to perform minor surgical procedures if necessary. The chiropodist can also advise you about your shoes (do not forget to ask about your running shoes as well). Some chiropodists like to see a pair of your older shoes when they assess you, so they can look at the way in which your walking has worn or rubbed them. Diabetics have priority access to chiropody in some Health Authority Districts.

Wound care specialist nurse

At present, few diabetes teams have a wound care nurse. She has received specialist training in the causes and assessment of ulcers and other skin conditions and in their treatment. Some people with diabetes have foot or leg ulcers and it is a considerable help to them to be able to see a wound care nurse regularly. There is some overlap between the role of the wound care nurse and the chiropodist and the latter will treat and dress foot ulcers too, if necessary.

Ophthalmologist, optometrist or ophthalmic optician

Some teams work with doctors who specialise in eye problems (ophthalmologists). Occasionally an optometrist or an ophthalmic optician will join the team. They are not doctors but have training in assessing your vision, the state of your eyes and in providing a prescription for glasses if necessary. All of these professionals will examine the back of your eye with a special magnifying torch called an ophthalmoscope. Diabetics are entitled to a free eye examination from an optometrist or ophthalmic optician once a year.

Psychologist

A few diabetes teams have regular contact with a clinical psychologist. Some people with diabetes have difficulty coming to terms with their condition, others may have pre-existing psychological difficulties which make it difficult to care for their diabetes. Many people have temporary ups and downs in their life with diabetes. If your problems are interfering with your life you may find some sessions with a psychologist helpful.

A psychologist is someone who studies and treats the variations of the way in which the normal human mind works and the way in which people behave. (A psychiatrist is a doctor who treats abnormalities or illnesses of the mind.)

A DIABETES SERVICE

This can mean your GP and his practice nurse working closely together and providing your diabetes care (using the resources of the hospital laboratory and working with a local chiropodist and dietician), or it can mean a hospital-based service. Or it often means both, working closely together.

This is an example of how one person was cared for:

John is 73 years old. Last year he saw his GP because of thirst and passing a lot of urine. Dr Jones tested his blood glucose and found that he had diabetes. Dr Jones runs a diabetic clinic at her surgery, and with the help of a dietician who comes once a month and the practice nurse, John's diabetes was well-controlled for a year. Dr Jones also arranged regular chiropody at the Community clinic. One week the chiropodist found that John had rubbed his toe on a new pair of shoes. It was ulcerated and badly infected. He cleaned it and dressed it and sent John straight to see Dr Jones. Dr Jones was worried about the infected toe so she telephoned the consultant diabetologist at the local hospital. He suggested that John come to the diabetic clinic at the hospital that day.

The diabetic clinic list was already full but anyone with an urgent problem is always seen. The receptionist was expecting John and the records clerk had made a new set of notes ready for him. The chiropodist worked there too so he brought John in to see the consultant diabetologist, Dr Smith. Together they examined John's foot very carefully. John had a bad infection which was spreading up the foot. There was evidence of diabetic nerve damage and the circulation was poor. The consultant explained to John that he needed urgent treatment in hospital including intravenous antibiotics and more detailed assessment of his foot.

John was admitted that day and interviewed and examined in detail by Dr Smith's house officer, and then by his registrar. His foot was X-rayed, swabbed, cleaned and dressed. He had blood tests and other investigations to check his general health. His blood glucose was very high because of the infection so he was given insulin treatment as well as the antibiotics.

That evening the vascular surgeon came to see him to assess his circulation and arranged an X-ray of the arteries in his legs. That was done next day and showed a narrowed artery which was improved there and then by a procedure called angioplasty. The circulation to the foot improved and slowly the infection settled.

While in hospital John was seen by the diabetic sister, had a revision session with the dietician and was given physiotherapy to keep his muscles strong while he was resting his foot. The wound care sister advised the ward nurses about dressing his toe. He got to know the whole medical team – Dr Smith, his registrar, senior house officer and house officer – because they saw him often.

After three weeks the foot was much better and John was ready to go home. Dr Smith's house officer telephoned Dr Jones to explain all that had happened and what the plan was now. She also gave John a letter for Dr Jones. John was back on his diabetes tablets again and the diabetic sister visited him at home to make sure that his blood glucose remained normal. He saw the wound care sister once a week to dress the healing ulcer on his toe and she liaised with the district nurse who came in daily. Dr Jones checked John's progress regularly. A month after his discharge from hospital John saw Dr Smith and the vascular surgeon in the out-patient clinic. The toe ulcer was now healed and the foot was back to normal. The chiropodist had ordered special shoes to protect John's feet in future and John found them very comfortable.

Now Dr Jones sees John at the diabetic clinic in the surgery every two months but shares his care with Dr Smith at the hospital. Other members of the diabetes team see him at intervals. To make sure that there is no confusion John carries a booklet in which all the health care professionals write their findings. He shows it to each of them when he sees them and keeps a close eye on his own progress.

Using your diabetes service

The keys to the service will be:

- Your doctor's name;
- His telephone number (day and emergency);
- Your doctor's timetable (and his receptionist's/secretary's);
- Your diabetes specialist nurse's name;
- Her telephone number (day and emergency);
- Your number (e.g. NHS number, hospital record number);
- The name of your diabetic clinic;
- The time and day on which it is held (it may not be weekly);

- The appointment system's rules (and arrangements for emergencies)

Hospital and surgery switchboards can be extremely busy. Make certain that you have dialled the right number and wait comfortably. They will answer eventually. Never be put off by switchboard operators or receptionists. Be polite but firm. If you need help, insist on getting it. (But if you feel really ill, call your GP to see you at home or dial 999.) Find out if there is a directly dialled telephone number rather than the main switchboard – it may be much quicker.

Remember that the operator will need to know exactly who you want. Also have your hospital number and consultant's name to hand – virtually all departments will ask for these. You will need your GP's name and any practice number when you telephone the surgery – large group practices deal with thousands of patients.

When you make contact, remind the person you are calling who you are. Do not be upset if he does not recollect all your details. It is not that he does not care, it is just that all health care professionals are very busy. I may see 60–100 patients a week, for example. The nurse or doctor will need to know who you are, a memory nudge about where and for what they see you, and a brief summary of why you are telephoning – for example:

'Hello, Sister Brown, it's Mrs Plunkett from Wimbledon. I come to the diabetic clinic. I saw you three weeks ago when I came for my routine check-up and everything was fine. But now my sugar is high even though I've increased my insulin. I take Mixtard twice a day. I don't feel ill. What should I do now?'

'Hello, Mrs Plunkett. I remember seeing you – you had just come back from Majorca, hadn't you. I'll pop in on my way home and we can look at your glucose levels together.'

Another practical point is to make sure that the details in your hospital and GP surgery records are correct. If your name or address are wrong you may be the subject of dangerous confusion or never receive letters or appointments. Make sure the computer has it right. Many hospitals use sticky labels for blood forms and other identification. If you move or discover an error ask staff to check that all the details in your records are right.

170

Help your doctor

'How is your diabetes, Mrs Green?' 'Well, its a bit up and down.' 'Do you mean your sugar levels are up and down?' 'Yes, I don't know why.' 'Please can I see your diabetes diary?' 'Sorry, I left it at home.' 'Well, can you remember any of your sugar values?' 'Oh, up and down, you know . . .' 'Have you changed your insulin?' 'No, I wasn't sure what to do.' 'Well, what insulin are you taking?' 'I don't know.' 'You don't know the name?' 'No, its in a bottle . . .'

This sort of exchange is not uncommon. Mrs Green's doctor is doing his best to help her but it is impossible without clearer information. Please help the health care professionals to help you.

SUMMARY

To gain most from the health care professionals who help you to care for your diabetes:

- Learn who they are, what they do and how to contact them.
- Learn how the diabetes service in your area works.
- Make sure that registration information is accurate.
- If you need help be polite but firm, ensure that staff know who you are and what the problem is.
- Help the diabetes team to help you.

16

PREGNANCY

Women with diabetes can have normal, healthy pregnancies and healthy babies. You will have to take a little more care of yourself than non-diabetic women, even before you become pregnant.

PLAN YOUR PREGNANCY

If you have diabetes it is important to ensure that you become pregnant only when you and your partner want to start a family. This is partly because unsuspected pregnancy could upset your glucose balance (see page 118), but more importantly because babies need a perfect environment in which to develop and grow in the womb. This means that the body chemicals to which the baby is exposed must be within normal limits. Unless the blood sugar is normal from the moment of conception, there is a risk of the baby's development being impaired or, rarely, of malformation.

But how can you tell the moment at which your baby is conceived? Most women do not realise they are pregnant until they have missed a period, and by then the baby has already been growing in the womb for several weeks. In order to be sure that your baby has the best start in life, decide with your partner when you want to become pregnant, use contraception and work on ensuring that your blood glucose is normal, and then stop the contraception.

The British Diabetic Association provides a lot of information about diabetes and pregnancy. Send for it straight away.

Contraception

As soon as a little girl has her first period, she is capable of bearing children. This means that mothers of diabetic girls should make sure that their daughters fully understand the facts of life. Ask your diabetes sister or doctor to help you if you find it difficult to discuss sexual matters. As soon as a diabetic woman starts to have sexual intercourse she should use contraception every time, except when she wants to become pregnant. As you are capable of child-bearing for 30 or more years the ideal method is one which does not expose your body to any risks, nor upsets your diabetes. The simplest methods are therefore barriers to sperm and spermicides. However, it is important that each couple uses the method which suits them and follows the instructions exactly. Barrier methods are effective only if used by people who take care to use them properly. The Pill only works if you take it precisely according to instructions. The rhythm method is not reliable and is inappropriate for diabetic women.

Condoms Condoms (or French letters) with spermicidal coating, cream or foam are best. They will not upset your diabetes, can be used easily any time and protect you and your partner from sexually exchanged disorders (including AIDS and gonorrhoea). If you have thrush or other minor fungal infections they may be passed on through intercourse, although they can occur in anyone, and be unrelated to sexual intercourse. Condoms may also reduce the risk of cervical cancer. The other advantage is that they are widely available in shops in Britain and easy to carry. They are less reliable than oral contraceptives, but the difference is small when condoms and spermicide are used together properly.

Diaphragms Diaphragms or Dutch caps have to be fitted for your vagina and you need to learn how to use them. Spermicidal cream is used with them. Once in place over the cervix they can be forgotten (although more spermicide is needed if you have intercourse more than once). They need to be removed and cleaned 6–8 hours after intercourse and some women find that they have more frequent urinary tract infections and vaginal discharge when using a diaphragm. They protect your cervix from sperm but you and your partner are not protected from infection.

Intra-uterine contraceptive devices IUCDs or coils can be used in diabetic women but there is a risk of pelvic infection which may, rarely, cause infertility. For this reason they are not very popular in

173

women whose diabetes makes them infection-prone.

Progestogen-only pills Otherwise known as 'mini-pills', these are the oral contraceptive of choice in diabetic women who insist on using the Pill. They have only a small risk of upsetting the blood glucose or blood fat balance. They have to be taken continuously (i.e. there should be no break during the fourth week of your menstrual cycle) – take your Pill with your insulin every day. Progestogen-only pills may temporarily suppress the periods altogether or cause erratic bleeding. They are slightly less effective than combined Pills.

Combined oral contraceptive pills with low dose oestrogen These can be used in diabetic women who are unable to use barrier methods reliably or dislike them. They carry a risk of blood clots, raised blood pressure, heart problems, stroke, and worsening of blood glucose balance and blood fats in any woman, but these side-effects are more likely in diabetic women, especially if you smoke or are overweight. Oral contraceptives are the most effective means of preventing pregnancy.

Morning after contraception Contraception in the form of a specific combined oral contraceptive can be given up to 72 hours after unprotected intercourse. See your doctor or a family-planning clinic as soon as possible if you have had a split condom or other problems with your usual contraception, or have had intercourse with no protection and do not want to become pregnant.

Sterilisation This should be regarded as irreversible but may be an option for men or women once you have completed your family. In a few instances, women with extremely severe diabetic tissue damage may be offered sterilisation as pregnancy would put them at risk.

Do we want a baby?

The decision to have a family needs a little thought if either parent has diabetes. Your children are more likely to develop diabetes than those of a non-diabetic couple. The risk of diabetes developing in your children is hard to calculate exactly – it depends on your country of origin, where you live now, your family history and many other factors. 0.35 per cent of the population have insulin-dependent diabetes. If both parents have insulin-dependent diabetes 30 per cent of their children may develop diabetes; if the father has diabetes the risk is 6 per cent; and if the mother has diabetes the risk is 1 per cent.

1–2 per cent of the population have non-insulin dependent diabetes. If both parents have diabetes 75 per cent of their children will eventually develop diabetes. If one parent has diabetes 15 per cent of their offspring will develop diabetes.

Although most people with diabetes who are planning a family will not have significant diabetic tissue damage, if you do have, especially if it is the woman who has diabetic complications, you need to consider whether you will be fit enough to go through pregnancy or to bring up a child. Pregnancy may worsen diabetic complications, especially eye and kidney disease. Discuss this with your doctor. Diabetic complications are not necessarily a bar to pregnancy, but you will need specialist advice and very intensive supervision.

What blood glucose level should I aim for?

Normal. All the time. As blood glucose balance is different in pregnancy compared with the non-pregnant state, this means blood glucose concentrations between 4 and 6 mmol/l (72–108 mg/dl).

Measure your blood glucose before each meal, before bed and after your largest meal of the day. Do this every day until the baby is born. Adjust your insulin every three or four days if necessary to achieve your target blood glucose.

Such tight blood glucose control means that you are at a greater risk of hypoglycaemia. Make sure you always have a bed-time snack to avoid night-time hypoglycaemia. Keep glucagon (see page 108) by you at home and teach your partner how to use it. Always carry your diabetic card and some glucose.

DIABETES TREATMENT DURING PREGNANCY

Adhere carefully to your diabetic diet (see the dietician for advice). Before pregnancy lose weight if you need to, but once pregnant do not starve yourself – it is not good for your baby.

It is unusual for women of child-bearing age to be taking glucose-lowering pills for their diabetes. If you are taking glucose-lowering pills your doctor will change you to insulin – this is because it allows more flexible and better glucose control and because of a possible risk of fetal malformation on pills.

Your insulin needs may fluctuate in the early stages of pregnancy, but as the weeks pass you will need more and more insulin. Keep increasing the dose according to your blood glucose levels, in close liaison with your diabetes team. By the end of pregnancy you may be taking twice your pre-pregnant insulin dose.

Care in pregnancy

When planning pregnancy ask if your local diabetes centre has a womens' diabetic clinic or a pre-pregnancy clinic. As soon as you suspect you are pregnant see your doctor. Pregnancy testing kits bought in chemists are usually very sensitive and accurate if used properly. However, remember that pregnancy tests may be negative in the very early stages of pregnancy – a blood test can confirm it. If in doubt assume you are pregnant.

Pregnant women with diabetes should be cared for by an obstetrician and a diabetologist working closely together. Find out if there is a special pregnancy diabetic clinic near you. Helping a diabetic woman through pregnancy is hard work for everyone – especially the mother-to-be. You will need to test your blood glucose and adjust your insulin carefully. You need extra ultrasound scans to check your baby's progress (some centres check special fetal heart scans routinely). There will be frequent visits to the antenatal clinics or pregnancy diabetic clinic. The reason for all this care is that diabetic women are more prone to the complications of pregnancy in addition to those of their diabetes. For example your blood pressure may rise, you may develop excess fluid around your baby. Your baby's growth is monitored very carefully because he may grow too big or not fast enough. In addition to the pregnancy checks you should have your eyes and kidney function checked at the beginning of pregnancy and later.

Delivery

This is always in a hospital with a special care baby unit in case your baby needs monitoring after birth (most hospitals do this routinely). There are differences of opinion as to when and how to deliver babies of diabetic mothers. Some centres allow women to go the full forty weeks if the baby is developing normally and the mother is well. Vaginal delivery is best provided the mother's pelvis is the right size and there are no problems with mother or baby. However, many obstetricians prefer to deliver the baby at about 37 or 38 weeks and would have a low threshold for caesarean section to ensure that the baby has no problems during labour. Discuss the options with your obstetrician – your treatment must be tailored to you and your baby.

While you are in labour you will have an intravenous drip with

176

glucose in it and insulin (if necessary) adjusted to your blood glucose level. This way you can have the energy and insulin you need finely tuned for you. As soon as the placenta is delivered your insulin requirements will fall to your pre-pregnant levels. It is very important that you remember this to avoid hypoglycaemia. You may stay in hospital a little longer than your non-diabetic friends.

Your baby may need extra glucose for the first day or so as he becomes used to life away from the diabetic womb. Previously babies of diabetic mothers were often large red cherubs. This is less common with good glucose balance in pregnancy. Occasionally he may have breathing problems. This is why it is important that there are facilities for special care of the newborn where your baby is born.

Home again

All the hard work in pregnancy is worthwhile when you take your new baby home. At this time you can relax your blood glucose control a little. You do not want to become hypoglycaemic while you are caring for a baby so aim for 6–8 mmol/l (108–144 mg/dl). Eat three meals and three snacks (you may find you need a midnight snack if your baby often gets you up at night). If you are breast feeding you may need more carbohydrate and may also need to adjust your insulin. Make sure you drink plenty. Try not to put on weight.

But what about father?

With all this attention focused on your wife you may feel a little left out. But it is very important that you share in the pregnancy throughout as your partner will need a great deal of support. If you do not already know how to do blood glucose tests, learn so that you can help her. Learn how to give insulin so that you can help with injections if necessary. And, very important, learn your partner's early warning signs for hypoglycaemia so that you can encourage her to eat glucose if necessary. Make sure that you have some glucagon (page 108) available in case she is unable to eat when hypo. Studies have shown that persistently high glucose levels are much more likely to harm the baby than hypoglycaemia, but it is still important to treat hypos promptly. Night-time hypoglycaemia seems particularly common during pregnancy – if your partner's breathing is unusual, she seems to be having a bad dream, is thrashing around or is sweating a lot, wake her and give glucose if appropriate. But you do not need to stay awake all night watching!

The frequent clinic visits can become tiring so try to help with transport if you can. Although diabetic women should not find pregnancy any more tiring than non-diabetics, the extra hassle may take its toll, so help at home with housework and any other children is always appreciated. Stress can upset diabetes so your partner needs a relaxing home environment at this time. You do too. It can be hard to strike the balance between helping your partner to keep an eye on her diabetes and general health and becoming overanxious. Discuss any concerns with the diabetes and antenatal team or your own doctor.

SUMMARY

- Women with diabetes can have healthy pregnancies and healthy babies.
- Pregnancy should be planned.
- Use contraception if you do not want to become pregnant.
- Barrier is best (if used properly).
- Keep your blood glucose level between 4 and 6 mmol/l (72–108 md/dl) from before pregnancy until delivery.
- Beware hypoglycaemia.
- Tell your doctor immediately you suspect you may be pregnant.
- Pregnancy is hard work for a diabetic woman, but the rewards are infinite.
- Don't forget dad!

17

SPORT AND EXERCISE

People with diabetes can enjoy most sports and other physical activities – and may excel in them.

EXERCISE IS GOOD FOR YOU

Exercise is good for everyone – it helps to keep your body trim and to keep your weight normal. It helps to strengthen your heart and lungs. It also improves your sensitivity to insulin and hence, your glucose tolerance. Regular exercise – by which I mean 20–30 minutes, at least three times a week, within the training zone (see page 182) – reduces your risk of having a heart attack. Exercise is good relaxation and most people who exercise regularly will also tell you it makes them feel good.

FUEL FOR EXERCISE

Body movement is produced by muscles. Different muscle groups contract and relax to produce different movements. Muscles contract and relax as you exercise. They need fuel to contract. The body supplies this in the bloodstream as glucose and fatty acids (produced from fat). The glucose and the fatty acids have to enter the muscle cells to provide the energy for contraction. Muscles store some glucose as glycogen – so this is used up when you first start to exercise. Soon your muscles need more fuel. You need a small amount of insulin to allow glucose and fatty acids into the muscle cells.

In a non-diabetic, as glucose leaves the bloodstream and the blood glucose level falls, the pancreas shuts off insulin production. This allows the liver to release glucose from its stores. Similarly, fatty acids can now be released from fat stores. So the blood glucose level does not fall below normal unless someone runs a marathon, or participates in some other endurance event. Glucose also arrives in the blood-stream from digestion of carbohydrate food in the gut.

In someone with insulin-treated or sulphonylurea-treated diabetes, glucose and fatty acids can enter the muscle cells, because there is usually plenty of insulin around. However, insulin production cannot be turned off as the blood glucose levels fall. High insulin levels prevent the liver from releasing glucose from its stores, and fatty acids cannot be released from body fat. But the muscles keep taking more and more glucose from the bloodstream, and the blood glucose level falls lower and lower. Eventually, you will become hypoglycaemic – unless you have eaten some glucose which is absorbed from the gut into the bloodstream. Other carbohydrate food will also eventually be absorbed as glucose – but more slowly because it has to be digested first.

So how do you exercise if you have diabetes and have no internal control over insulin production? It is not as critical as it seems. If you are planning new or vigorous exercise, reduce the insulin (e.g. by 10–50 per cent of your usual dose) or reduce your pills (e.g. by half a pill) which will be acting at that time. Eat more long-acting carbohydrate (i.e. high-fibre, starchy carbohydrate) at the meal before, and have some glucose immediately before exercising, and if necessary during exercise (e.g. at half-time). After exercising have some more long-acting carbohydrate. Check your blood glucose levels before and after (if necessary during) your exercise and use this information to work out what to do next time. Your diabetes adviser will be able to help you.

A word of warning. Do not exercise vigorously with a high glucose, especially if you have ketones in your urine. If you have no insulin in the circulation, exercise will push your blood glucose up further as the liver releases glucose but the muscles cannot use it. Fatty acids cannot be used either and the liver breaks them down into ketones. This makes your blood acid. You would eventually develop diabetic ketoacidosis (page 99). Give yourself some insulin to return the glucose towards normal (but not hypoglycaemic) and wait for it to work. It is better not to exercise vigorously that day if you can avoid it but to allow your diabetes control to improve. This can also happen if you overeat before or during exercise.

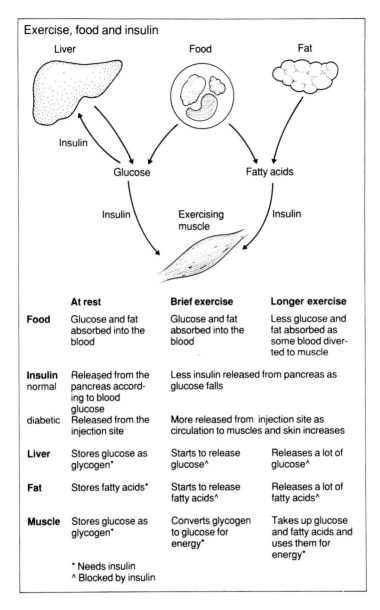

Exercise, food and insulin

Liver   Food   Fat

Insulin

Glucose   Fatty acids

Insulin   Exercising muscle   Insulin

	At rest	**Brief exercise**	**Longer exercise**
Food	Glucose and fat absorbed into the blood	Glucose and fat absorbed into the blood	Less glucose and fat absorbed as some blood diverted to muscle
Insulin normal	Released from the pancreas according to blood glucose	Less insulin released from pancreas as glucose falls	
diabetic	Released from the injection site	More released from injection site as circulation to muscles and skin increases	
Liver	Stores glucose as glycogen*	Starts to release glucose^	Releases a lot of glucose^
Fat	Stores fatty acids*	Starts to release fatty acids^	Releases a lot of fatty acids^
Muscle	Stores glucose as glycogen*	Converts glycogen to glucose for energy*	Takes up glucose and fatty acids and uses them for energy*

* Needs insulin
^ Blocked by insulin

Exercise, food and insulin

FIT TO EXERCISE?

Before starting an exercise programme discuss what you are planning to do with your doctor. Virtually everyone can exercise but if you have heart problems or muscle or joint problems you may need to choose the form and vigour of your exercise carefully. If you have just had laser treatment for retinopathy or a vitreous haemorrhage you should not exercise until given the all-clear by your doctor. You must not do exercises which could knock, rub or put pressure on a foot or leg ulcer.

As a general rule, never exercise so energetically that you cannot hold a conversation with someone while exercising. Learn how to take your pulse at the wrist. The pulse rate should not exceed the maximum rate for your age. The pulse rate at rest is about 60 to 80 beats a minute. Your training rate should be 60–85 per cent of your maximum. You can calculate this by subtracting your age in years from 220. Thus for a 50-year-old man the maximum heart rate is 220 − 50 = 170 beats per minute. His training rate is 120–144 beats per minute which should be sustained for 20–30 minutes each week for maximum benefit. If you do not exercise regularly start at the 60 per cent end (102 beats per minute in this case), and work up towards 85 per cent (144 beat/min) over several weeks or months.

Work up to it gently. There is no point finishing your first exercise session drenched in sweat and gasping for air with an impression of imminent demise. Next morning your continued existence will be made only too plain by the discovery of muscles you didn't know you had, none of which now work and all of which ache abominably. The end result is a fervent determination never to exercise again! Warm up first with some gentle loosening-up exercises and then begin a graded

Training zone for exercise

Your age in years	Your heart rate in beats per minute	
	60% maximum	85% maximum
20	120	170
30	114	161
40	108	153
50	102	144
60	96	136
70	90	127

programme which suits your own fitness level and needs. Stretch those stiff muscles and joints carefully. If it hurts don't do it. Wind down gently at the end.

Ask your doctor's advice on exercising safely *before* you start – not while he is treating your tennis elbow!

SPORT FOR ALL

There are hundreds of sporting activities to choose from, but you do not need to take up an organised sport. Walking in your favourite countryside, energetic gardening can all give you regular exercise. But if you decide to take up a particular sport, how do you decide whether you, as a person with diabetes can do it? I wrote these guidelines for this book and modified them following very helpful discussions with co-members of the BDA Sports and Exercise Working Party.

Can I do this activity?

How fit am I?

- You should always discuss exercise with your doctor.
- Is your exercise tolerance good? (Can you walk upstairs easily, run for a bus, mow the lawn for example?)
- Has your doctor told you to avoid any activities?
- Do you have diabetic eye disease, foot problems, heart disease or other diabetic tissue damage? If yes, discuss exercise with your doctor.
- Following a heart attack you should avoid vigorous exercise for two months limiting your exercise to walking.
- People with active new vessel disease of the eye should avoid excessive exertion until the eyes have been adequately treated. If you exercise too strenuously it can precipitate a bleed from these new vessels into the eye.
- If you have foot ulcers you should avoid weight bearing altogether on the affected foot. If you have a poor nerve supply or poor blood supply to your feet you should, in addition, have your feet checked regularly by a state registered chiropodist.

Is my blood glucose balance safe?

- Is my blood glucose under control?
- Do you know how to adjust your diet and treatment for different

exercise levels? If not, ask your diabetes adviser.

- Do you take insulin or pills which may cause hypoglycaemia? If so, can you recognise and treat hypoglycaemia?
- Do you have hypoglycaemia often or without warning? If yes, consult your diabetes adviser.

Can I do this particular exercise safely?

- Does it involve short bursts of activity or prolonged, endurance exertion?
- Can you eat, take your treatment (if necessary) and test your blood glucose during the exercise?
- Can you keep food and diabetes equipment with you and have you planned what to do if you become hypoglycaemic?
- How easy would it be for you to predict your energy expenditure and plan your eating and treatment before, during and after exercise?
- If the activity is done outdoors what would happen if you needed assistance? Are you alone or with others? Are you close to a telephone or transport?
- Does it involve heat or cold, heights or depths, water or air? All of these can influence your blood glucose balance in addition to the exercise.

Is this sport or activity suitable for me?

There are regulations for some sports which relate to people with diabetes. The BDA has a list of most of them. Ask your doctor whether he thinks this sport is appropriate for you.

This may seem a formidable list, but remember it is designed to include 70 year olds as well as teenagers. Most of my readers will have no problems learning the majority of sports and will require this list only when contemplating unknown or potentially hazardous activities. Providing you learn from the experts and observe safety rules carefully, people with diabetes can take up sports such as rock-climbing or slalom canoeing. Tim, with newly-diagnosed diabetes, learned to climb on a BDA/Outward Bound mountain course, sought further training, put in a great deal of practice and, a year later, climbed the Old Man of Hoy – a 500 foot stack of rock towering above dangerous seas. But you do not have to opt for such dramatic activities. Choose one that interests you.

Disabilities such as amputations or blindness are no barrier to most

184

sports. I have met people who are wheelchair-bound who go canoeing and even abseiling. I also know a blind man who has just scaled Mont Blanc and enjoys a range of sports including water-skiing and judo. And several people whose vision has been severely impaired have successfully completed Outward Bound mountain courses with me at Eskdale.

THE PERSON SUPERVISING THE ACTIVITY

If a sports instructor is unfamiliar with diabetes it may help to go through the following list with him. Suggest he asks himself the following questions.

Can a person with diabetes do it safely?

- Do you understand what diabetes is and what it means? Are you aware of the different types of diabetes and their treatment?
- Are there regulations about people with diabetes doing this activity – do they apply here?
- The main risks are hypoglycaemia and the effects of tissue damage (the latter are covered in the section for people with diabetes, page 183). Do you understand what hypoglycaemia is and how you may recognise it? (See page 101). Hypoglycaemia, which some-times causes confusion or coma, may not only affect the indi-vidual, but others involved in the activity, bystanders and those involved in rescue.
- If the person becomes hypoglycaemic will he be a danger to himself or others? If yes, will he and you be able to recognise the warning symptoms, and will he be able to eat and cure the hypoglycaemia? If he does become seriously hypoglycaemic can you safeguard him (and others) and treat/rescue him if required?

Can this person with diabetes do it safely?

- Is he physically and mentally fit enough to start this activity?
- Have you gone through pages 183 and 184 with the person?
- Can he adjust his diabetic treatment and diet to enjoy this activity safely without losing control of his diabetes?

Can I supervise him?

- Do I, personally, feel competent to supervise him in this activity? Will I need additional help?

- It is natural to worry about looking after someone with a medical condition with which you are unfamiliar – but diabetes is no barrier to performing well in most activities – sometimes at national or international level. Some sporting bodies do have regulations banning people with diabetes who take insulin. However, many have no clear policy. Most national diabetes associations will advise people with diabetes and sporting organisations. The British Diabetic Association in liaison with the Sports Council is collecting information on a wide range of activities and the regulations if any, and will be pleased to help both sports trainers and sportsmen and women.

COMMON PROBLEMS

Preventing hypoglycaemia

Reduce your insulin or sulphonylurea pills, eat enough fast and slow carbohydrate and test your glucose. It is as simple as this, but may be a little more difficult in practice.

Reduce your insulin or pills How much should you reduce your insulin? It is usually enough to reduce it by 2–4 units, but some people may need to halve the dose of the insulin which will be acting at the time of the activity. Thus for a morning activity, reduce your morning fast-acting insulin. For an afternoon activity reduce your lunch-time fast-acting or your morning medium-acting insulin. For an evening activity reduce your evening short-acting. You may also wish to reduce your evening medium or long-acting insulin a little to reduce the risk of nocturnal hypoglycaemia. For regular vigorous activity reduce your total insulin dose by at least 20 per cent.

As an approximate guide, reduce the dose of pills taken before the exercise by a quarter to a third of your usual total daily dose.

Eat more You need slow, starchy, high-fibre carbohydrate to last you through the exercise and to help you recover in the hours afterwards. You need glucose for rapid energy, that will provide a boost when you want it. As a rough guide, double the carbohydrate in the last meal before vigorous exercise, have one and half times normal before moderate exercise. Have a double snack before strenuous exercise, or replace the snack with a Mars bar or equivalent – miniMars for moderate exercise, full-size for energetic exercise. Slip in some glucose as tablets or drink if you feel low during the exercise.

'But I want to slim', you wail! So, greatly reduce your insulin or sulphonylurea pills before exercise and keep a very close eye on your blood glucose levels. People on metformin alone do not need to worry about eating extra before exercise; hypoglycaemia is most unlikely and most people on metformin alone usually have a weight problem so more food is not a good idea.

As you become familiar with a particular activity, you will be able to fine-tune your insulin and food. Most people who exercise regularly will not need large increases in their food.

Measure your blood glucose Do this often to start with and then as needed. It is the key to success. Blood glucose testing has freed people with diabetes from anxiety about the effects of exercise and other experiences upon their diabetes. Don't worry about your glucose – test it and establish the facts. Then you can learn from each training session.

TYPES OF EXERCISE

Sprinting

This uses the glycogen stored in your muscles. Some people eat plenty of carbohydrate in the days before an event to top-up muscle stores. You will probably not want a lot in your stomach immediately before racing, so make sure you eat a meal high in starchy fibrous carbohydrate earlier in the day. Some people may take some neat glucose as a non-fizzy drink, tablets or gel just before running to start topping-up your bloodstream and thus your muscles once the muscle glycogen has been used up by the sprint. It may be difficult to eat right away because the intensive exercise can make people feel a little nauseous or cramped. Eat when you have finished. Again train gradually and learn how much carbohydrate loading to do beforehand and how much insulin or tablets and food to take that day as you train.

Endurance exercise

This includes marathon running and walking. You will soon use up your muscle glycogen stores and start drawing glucose out of the bloodstream so you not only need to eat beforehand but to keep topping up as you go along. Unless you have got your insulin or pill dose exactly right, you may have too much insulin around to allow your liver to release glucose when you need it. Reduce your insulin or sulphonylurea pills by 50 per cent when you start training if you have never walked or run a long way before. If you have trained you will be able gradually to work out how much to take. What you eat as you go along depends on the type of exercise and how competitive it is. Fluids and electrolytes are important, especially so if you are running, and/or it is hot, and your glucose top-ups can be part of your drinks. Walkers can browse on fruit and nuts, biscuits and muesli bars with the occasional chocolate bar for emergency energy. For a day's strenuous walking with a heavy rucksack you need three big meals with plenty of starchy high fibre carbohydrate, and six double snacks (i.e. the carbohydrate equivalent of twelve of your normal snacks). Once you get into training you may manage on less but start off with this. Whether walking or running you must have some glucose with you in a pocket or hip/bum bag.

ENVIRONMENTAL HAZARDS

Water

Look at the second-hand on your watch. Take a deep breath in and hold it. How long can you hold your breath for? That is the length of time you have to sort yourself out if you get into difficulties under-water. This is the most hazardous environment for the hypogly-caemia-prone diabetic. This is also why under-water diving is not a safe sport for most people taking insulin. A few, entirely confident in their knowledge of diabetes self-care and their freedom from hypo-glycaemia, do dive. With any water sport it is essential that you do not become hypoglycaemic while on, in or under the water. It is rare for someone to become unconscious from hypoglycaemia (see page 106) but this could be disastrous while swimming or canoeing. Follow the rules for all exercise, but I would also suggest 2–4 glucose tablets just before setting off or entering the water. This means that you will be exercising on a rising glucose. Never go on/in water alone and always wear a life jacket or buoyancy aid or swim where there is a lifeguard. A wet suit alone is not enough – it will not always keep your head above water if you become unconscious. On boating or canoe trips keep snacks in a water-proof container tied into the boat. Rowing is one of the most strenuous sports there is and often requires both sprint and endurance effort. You must stoke up with enormous amounts of carbohydrate. In this sport the rest of the eight will not be pleased if you break stroke to eat half-way through a race!

When I checked Josephine's blood glucose before she got into her kayak, it was 13 mmol/l (234 mg/dl). She was an accomplished canoeist. Fifteen minutes later she was going round and round in erratic and uncoordinated circles. Her blood glucose was now 2 mmol/l (36 mg/dl). A bottle of Hypostop glucose gel revived her and after a couple of biscuits, she continued the session.

Hypostop glucose gel is useful for water activities. It comes in a leakproof polythene bottle and can be tied onto your clothing or pinned into a pocket. It is easy to take in water. One diabetic acquaintance who dives carries and eats Mars bars underwater. If you need to eat in unusual places practice first.

Large numbers of people with diabetes enjoy water sports safely and so can you if you wish. Learn from a recognised trainer and use some commonsense to prevent hypoglycaemia.

Heights

Most activities involving heights are safety-roped so they are often safer than water sports. Fear is a common factor for all of us at great heights and this causes adrenaline surges with racing heart, sweating and shaking – just like a hypo. If in doubt you must assume you are hypo and eat glucose. Rock climbing is a strenuous sport punctuated by periods of waiting.

Eat glucose just before you start climbing so that you are exercising on a rising glucose. If you are safeguarding someone else (e.g. on belay) you must be certain that you cannot become hypoglycaemic. As belaying takes two hands eat a Mars bar and some dextrosol *before* you tell the climber he or she can start climbing. (It is, of course, essential to tell your climbing partner that you have diabetes and unforgiveable to become hypoglycaemic when you have someone else's life in your hands.) People can become hypoglycaemic abseiling too – although fear should increase the glucose as emergency hormones are released, I have seen people become hypoglycaemic with fear. So, again eat glucose before you set off to ensure that your descent is as controlled as you would wish. People with diabetes go parachute jumping and hang-gliding – seek expert advice before tackling such hazardous sports. For any of these sports you must have some means of keeping glucose on your person no matter what position you end up in. The bum bag worn on the side or tum, with a zip at the top, is one way.

Depths

Caving or pot-holing may include some climbing and some water. In addition to these dangers, one of its main features is that you are inaccessible once deep in the cave system. You must be certain that you have enough to eat and plenty to spare for unexpected delays. As with hang-gliding, think carefully before taking yourself and your diabetes down a pot-hole.

COMPETITIVE AND TEAM SPORTS

If you are simply pursuing a sport on your own for pleasure you need not be under pressure to compare your performance with others and you will not be a member of a team who are relying on you to pull your weight.

> Joe and John were orienteering. They had to navigate and run a complex course competing against 10 other pairs and against the clock. There was a prize for the fastest team to find all the markers. Joe had diabetes. They jogged off and all was well to start with. They found the first two markers. Then they could not find the third. John started to get cross. 'We've slowed down, the others are catching up.' Then he noticed the landmark he had been looking for and raced towards it. Joe had been feeling slightly wobbly and was just getting some glucose tablets out of his bum bag. He tried to eat them as he ran after John and choked on the crumbs. Then he dropped the pack into some undergrowth. He stopped to look for it. John looked back. 'Come on, slow coach' he shouted, 'run, why are you stopping?'. Joe was feeling rather dizzy by now but he did not want to let John down and so he stumbled on up the hill. When he reached the top, panting, John was already racing downhill to the next marker. Joe followed. He was sweating and shaky and everything seemed very hazy. When Joe did not appear at the next marker, John went back to look for him and found him semi-conscious at the bottom of the hill where he had fallen. Fortunately after he was revived with a can of glucose drink he just had a few bruises.

Hypoglycaemia can induce a state of mind in which people do not want to stop what they are doing (see page 106). Furthermore, it is natural to ignore minor symptoms so as to avoid letting a friend or team mates down, especially when an event is timed. It is best to ensure that the hypo does not happen in the first place. But if it does, it is faster (and safer) in the long run to stop and deal with it, as continued exercise will make it worse. John knew that Joe had diabetes

190

and what to do to help him. Make sure your team mates know this. If you are playing professionally or in national competitions (as several people with diabetes do), you will have built up extensive experience of your exact treatment and food needs during training with the rest of the team. Use training to perfect your skills in the game and in diabetes management.

ACTIVITIES IN GENERAL

Most people who take part in activities are not involved in marathon running, rock climbing or team sports at national level. However, the sections above should help you to consider the safety aspects of any more usual activities in which you wish to participate.

SUMMARY

- Exercise is good for people with diabetes.

- Consult your doctor before starting exercise or sport.

- Learn how to exercise and train safely.

- Learn how to adjust your diet and treatment for exercise.

- Gain a realistic understanding of the potential dangers in any new sport and how to safeguard yourself and others.

- Plan ahead.

- Tell your team mates and instructors that you have diabetes.

- Train for your diabetes care as well as the activity and physical fitness. Learn by experience.

- Have a go with expert help.

18

TRAVEL

People with diabetes can and do travel all over the world. To ensure that your holiday or business trip is memorable for the right reasons put a little forethought into your travel arrangements. The following points are a general guide – choose those which are appropriate to your trip.

PLAN AHEAD

Where are you going?

Clearly a journey from Manchester to Birmingham is less complicated than an expedition to Tierra del Fuego. Are you going to a familiar place or breaking new ground? While there is no reason why someone with diabetes should not travel in remote mountains or in the depths of the rain forest, to do this you have to be very confident of your diabetes self-care if you are insulin-dependent. New diabetics may choose to spend your first holiday after diagnosis somewhere familiar or not too far off the beaten track. You are unlikely to have much choice in your destination with a business trip. A mystery tour (deliberate or unintentional) can be fun, but if you are taking glucose-lowering treatment with pills or insulin you may prefer to plan your route carefully to avoid unexpected delays or being stranded. It is always useful to learn how to read a map, if you do not already know.

Is a visa required? Do you need immunisations? If yes, have all of them, including any non-compulsory ones advised by your doctor. Sarah (page 53) had a high glucose for several days after her influenza immunisation – similar effects may occur with other immunisations so it is better to have them well before you travel. Always keep your tetanus shots up to date.

What language is spoken? Clearly it is easier visiting an English-speaking country. If you do not speak the language of the country you are visiting, it is wise to have a basic phrase book, or better to learn some words before you go. At the very least, learn the words for 'diabetes' 'insulin injection' (if necessary), 'help' and 'doctor'. Ensure that you have some small denomination local currency with you to buy food or make telephone calls if necessary. If you can afford it, carry enough money, travellers cheques or credit cards to get yourself home if an emergency arose.

When are you going?

How far ahead is your journey? Tomorrow? Or do you have time to plan? If you are someone whose job or hobby often takes you away from home at short notice, you must keep a diabetes travel pack ready to go. At what time of year is your journey? You need to consider the weather in your country of departure, and what the weather will be like when you get where you are going. Extremes of heat or cold, wet or dry, or high winds, can affect everyone's health; and may require special care with your diabetes equipment and insulin or tablets. (For example, insulin goes off if it overheats – see page 86. It does not work if it has been frozen. Blood-glucose testing strips must be kept dry or they will not produce accurate results.)

With whom are you travelling?

'I travel alone, sometimes I'm East, sometimes I'm West. No remem-bered love can ever find me.' Noel Coward enjoyed solitary travel. But if you have diabetes and get into difficulties – hypoglycaemia or gastroenteritis, for example – you may be very pleased to see your remembered love – or just a good friend. The choice is yours, but common sense suggests that, for prolonged trips or distant ones, people with diabetes are safer travelling with a companion. If you are travelling with other people you must tell them about your diabetes.

Patrick was on an initiative course with ten of his work-mates. They had been together for a week, trying a wide range of activities. The others noticed that Patrick did not look well, but he brushed their concern aside. 'I'm fine,' he said, 'Let's go and have a pint, I'm parched.' Patrick drank a lot – mostly beer. Next day the group set off on a two day exercise, navigating over the moor to a hut to sleep, then walking back to base. Patrick was soon at the back of the group, puffing and panting. The others asked if he was all right. 'A bit of a hangover,' said Patrick, ruefully. It took them a long time to reach the hut. Patrick vomited several times in the night. 'Bad beer,' he gasped. Next morning he was drowsy and clearly could not walk. After much anxious discussion, two of his friends stayed with him while the rest went for help. When the group's tutor and a rescue party opened the door, the whole hut smelled of rotten apples. They searched his rucksack and found some insulin and a glucose-testing kit. Fortunately for Patrick, the tutor's wife is diabetic. He realised what was wrong, checked Patrick's glucose – which was 44 mmol/l (792 mg/dl) on the strip and gave him some insulin. Then they took him to hospital. Patrick could have died from this episode of ketoacidosis.

If you are taking glucose-lowering therapy, tell your companions about hypoglycaemia and what to do about it. If you are prone to bad hypos, teach a close companion how to give glucagon (see page 108). If your friends know that you have diabetes, they will not wonder why you have special dietary needs. And you need not hide your blood testing from them.

How long?

Consider the duration of the journey itself and the length of the whole trip. During a long journey you will need to eat, and may need to check your glucose. You may travel across time zones, in which case many people find it easier to stay on home time until you arrive, and then change to foreign time. On the return trip, stay in foreign time until you reach your home country and time zone (see page 200).

Ensure that you have enough supplies to last the whole trip and to cover losses or breakages. Your doctor and chemist will need notice of your requirements, especially if you are going away for a long time.

How are you travelling?

This affects several aspects of your diabetes care. If you are travelling under your own steam – walking or cycling, for example, you need to fuel your exercise (see page 179). If you are using your own car you must follow all the driving rules (see page 157) and do not forget your Green Card, or other documentation if you are travelling abroad. With public transport you are completely dependent on others. A good general rule is to assume the worst – that the train will stop for no apparent reason in the middle of a featureless landscape for three

hours and cause you to miss your connection; or that your Mediter-
ranean holiday will terminate in a day and night at a small, hot airport
clutching a straw donkey, two funny-shaped bottles of potent local
spirit and a bag of olives (leaking) while your plane awaits a vital
component available only from the other side of the world. Your
planning (i.e. food, drink and treatment) should take such contingen-
cies into account. Sufferers from motion sickness should, if possible,
try to avoid the mode of travel most likely to precipitate this. People
with diabetes can take motion sickness pills if they wish. Follow the
dosage and precautions advised by your doctor or pharmacist.

Accommodation

Where will you be staying? In a hotel? A tent? Self-catering cottage?
Bed and Breakfast? Youth hostels? Obviously if you have a room to
yourself it will be easier to look after your diabetes in private. A fridge
will ensure that your insulin stays cool. If you are sharing with
strangers keep your diabetes kit secure – be particularly careful to lock
up your insulin and syringes. (This is another reason why an insulin
pen is simpler – you carry it with you – although you should still lock
away your back up supplies.)

Food

One of the joys of travelling is the opportunity to try exotic foods. Do
your best to stick to your diet, but do not worry if you cannot follow it
exactly. A good start is to find out about the country's staple
carbohydrate foods before you go. These include bread (i.e. pumper-
nickel, chapati, rye-bread, unleavened bread, corn-bread, nan, crisp-
bread, pitta), rice, potatoes, yams, pasta, sweet potato, cassava, maize,
porridge, plantain, lentils and beans. Fruit provides carbohydrate too.
Wash it well or peel it. To fill up there will always be local vegetables.
Most places will provide salad – but this must be well-washed and if
in doubt, you are better with cooked vegetables (or wash the salad
yourself). Choose grilled meat or fish if possible and avoid very fatty
meat or meat dishes such as paté fois gras. Eat cheese sparingly.
Avoid obviously sugary sweets and puddings.

Try local beverages if you wish, but do not overdo the alcohol. Use
bottled mineral water on which you break the seal if you are unsure
about the purity of tap water. Have some fruit juice if you wish, but
remember that it is often sugary.

As soon as you arrive find out hotel or bed and breakfast meal
times. Identify local restaurants and shops. Check opening hours of

shops, holy days, religious festivals, early closing etc. If you are on sulphonylurea drugs or insulin it is essential that you eat regularly. So do not be caught out. Always carry some energy rations (some countries – Australia for example – will not allow you to bring in certain types of food). Prepacked fibre crunch or muesli bars are easy to carry. Take some boxed or canned drink too.

Activity

What are you going to do while you are away? Lying on the beach uses less energy than tramping around ancient monuments. If your activity level is going to differ greatly from what you would do at home, adjust your diet and treatment to cope with this (see page 180). Do not be tempted into hazardous activities 'because we're on holiday' without giving them the same thought that you would at home. Are they properly supervised? How can you prevent yourself becoming hypoglycaemic.

Getting around

Local transport may be excellent or non-existent. It is all part of the adventure – your rickshaw may deliver you promptly from door-to-door or you may fail to decipher the hieroglyphics on the bus and end up ten miles in the wrong direction (I've done this in London!). Carry your diabetes kit and some food with you so that you do not need to worry if you are late back for a meal.

Local hazards

Without wishing to put you off, exotic travel can have a wide range of hazards. Bears, crocodiles, spiders, scorpions and assorted snakes spring to mind. But there are smaller dangers which may catch you unawares – malaria and other parasitic diseases. Always take your antimalarial prophylaxis exactly as instructed. Do not paddle in rivers or lakes in tropical countries. Be careful on the beach. Any small injury – a blister, cut or bite may become infected in hot countries so look after your skin very carefully and carry a first aid kit. Gastroenteritis is very common – avoid it (see page 202).

What happens if something goes wrong?

You must have full medical insurance. It should provide treatment while you are away and, if necessary, get you home with a medical escort if you become very ill abroad. The hospital in which I work

196

serves Heathrow airport. I see people with diabetes who have become ill abroad and who have been unable to find proper medical advice. They hang on getting iller and iller until their booked flight home. They struggle onto the plane and have a terrible journey often requiring help from other passengers. By the time they arrive they are dehydrated and collapsed and have to be rushed to hospital to be resuscitated.

Always check the small print very carefully as many insurance policies will not cover you for pre-existing illness. Be particularly careful with policies included in package holidays – you may need to ask your travel agent to show you the rules. Shop around – as with car insurance there are wide variations.

When you return

Carry on with your antimalarials. Keep your diabetes diary safely so that you can use it to plan another trip.

STEP BY STEP

BDA Travel Guide

The British Diabetic Association has good information on most countries, with Travel Guides including useful phrases in the language of the country concerned. Other national diabetes organisations may provide similar support. Send for your Travel Guide as soon as you know you are going.

Are you fit to go?

If you are in any doubt about your fitness ask your doctor *before* you book your ticket.

Booking

Tell the airline, hotel, travel company that you have diabetes. Some airlines will provide a diabetic diet if asked in advance. Many hotels will help. Your package tour organiser should know too. If you are elderly or have a physical difficulty wheelchairs can be provided at stations, ports and airports if you give advance warning.

Diabetes check-up

Before a long or very distant trip the following points should be checked.

- Glucose balance. What to do with treatment while travelling and while away, including emergencies.
- Tissue damage. Is there any and do you need to take any special precautions?
- Dietitian – for dietary advice.
- Chiropodist – for foot check and foot care advice.
- Doctor's letter to confirm that you have diabetes and the generic names of all medications. Note of allergies and other medical conditions.
- Supplies for your diabetes travel pack.

Diabetes travel pack

This should contain the following:

- Medic-alert or SOS medallion or bracelet (to be worn);
- Diabetic card;
- Letter from doctor confirming diabetes;
- Letter in language of country visited confirming diabetes;
- Treatment (take twice the amount you need)
  - insulin, syringes, needles, needle clipper
  - cool bag for insulin (4 to 25°C)
  - insulin pen, pen needles, insulin cartridges (plus a needle and syringe) or
  - glucose-lowering pills;
- Testing
  - blood testing strips (with meter or biosensor if used), finger-pricker, lancets, platforms if needed
  - urine testing strips for glucose and ketones
  - diabetic diary with pen;
- Hypoglycaemia treatment (if on sulphonylureas or insulin)
  - glucose tablets
  - hypostop
  - glucagon kit (if on insulin).

Medical kit

This should contain the following:

- Other medication;
- Antidiarrhoeal (e.g. codeine phosphate);
- Antibiotic (e.g. ampicillin or erythromycin if penicillin-allergic) if your doctor agrees;
- Motion sickness pills;
- Headache pills (e.g. paracetamol);
- Antiseptic wipes;
- Antiseptic cream;
- Assorted dressings;
- Roll of tape (e.g. Micropore);
- Foot care items from chiropodist;
- Non-adherent dressing (e.g. N-A dressing);
- Absorbent gauze;
- Triangular bandage;
- Open weave bandage;
- Eye pad;
- Safety pins (use nappy pins with protected ends);
- Round-ended tweezers;
- Round-ended scissors;
- Sunscreen cream;
- Thin foil space blanket;
- Torch;
- Paper tissues;
- Polythene bags.

NB Never use a safety pin next to the skin. Never put tape or bandages all the way around a toe or limb – it may constrict the circulation.

Out and about kit

- Diabetes travel pack;
- Plastic bottle of mineral water with screw top;
- Box(es) or can(s) of drink;
- Wholemeal biscuits or foil-wrapped fibre or muesli bars;
- Local money to put in pay phone;
- Selected items from your medical kit.

Packing

Protect yourself from extremes of temperature. But do not pack so much that your suitcase is too heavy to carry.

Remember that in some forms of transport your suitcase will be taken away and stowed in the hold. Keep your diabetes kit with you in your hand luggage. A shoulder bag is useful for your out and about kit. Some people like a bum bag or ski bag worn around the waist. It is possible to fit all your diabetes kit and your out and about kit (except the water) into a large bum bag.

Setting off

People whose diabetes is controlled on diet alone and most of those on tablet treatment will not need to make any special treatment adjustments for the day of travel, although those on sulphonylureas may wish to reduce their morning dose for a very long or arduous journey.

Not flying

For all but short journeys, if you take insulin injections, you should reduce your morning dose by 10 per cent. It is better to have blood glucose levels above 6 mmol/l (108 mg/dl) while travelling to avoid hypoglycaemia. Test your blood glucose before each full meal and before bed, or 4–6 hourly.

Flying on insulin

You may cross time zones. For short flights and if the time difference is less than four hours this rarely requires much change in your insulin. Just make sure you cannot become hypoglycaemic. For longer journeys consider the day of travel as a special day and resume your normal insulin at breakfast-time in the country to which you are travelling (by breakfast I mean their first meal in the morning). On the day of travel you may be awake for longer than usual whether or not it is night or day on the ground below. Add up the insulin you usually have in each 24 hours and use commonsense to make the suggested changes at an appropriate time of day. For example, on Westward flights, take extra fast-acting at extra meals after checking your blood glucose. On Eastward flights reduce your insulin.

Customs and security

You do not have to declare your diabetes at either of these points but with the current concern about drug smuggling, syringes and needles are likely to be commented upon if found in a routine search. This is no problem, but a note in the language of the country you are visiting can make explanations easier. (Some countries have the death penalty for drug smuggling.)

WHILE AWAY

Many people travel to experience something different from everyday life. This can include temperatures, humidity, terrain, sleeping/waking patterns, food and many other facets of life. Some of these could change your glucose balance.

Heat

Protect your skin from the sun.

Marie has diabetic neuropathy. She went on holiday to Italy. The sun blazed in a cloudless sky. Each morning she covered herself in sunscreen cream before going out. One day she paddled in the pool during the morning. By lunchtime her feet were scarlet. The blisters ruined her holiday and took a month to heal.

Hot weather also increases the circulation to your skin so your insulin may be absorbed more rapidly and may work earlier and more strongly than you expect.

Cold

This decreases the circulation to your skin as the body conserves its heat. Thus your insulin may be absorbed more slowly than you expect, only to appear later when you warm up. If your circulation is poor, especially in your feet, the circulation may be reduced to a critical level and you may lose the blood flow to your toes. Gangrene is a rare consequence. If you have poor circulation keep your feet well insulated from the cold.

Hypoglycaemia reduces your ability to shiver to keep warm. This means that if you become severely hypoglycaemic in cool weather your body temperature will fall. Once you have eaten and your blood glucose rises to normal you will start to shiver and warm up. This is a potentially dangerous problem in harsh environments. In this situation, anyone with diabetes who appears hypothermic must also be treated for hypoglycaemia, and anyone who is hypoglycaemic must also be treated for hypothermia.

201

Gastroenteritis

Sadly, many holidays include a day or so with Travellers' Tummy or Montezuma's Revenge. This is largely preventable by eating well-cooked food which has not been left standing, drinking bottled mineral or spring water, eating only well-washed salad and peeled fruit. If you do develop diarrhoea and/or vomiting, retire to bed near a toilet with some sealed bottles of water, some cans of Coca Cola or Pepsi Cola (they contain glucose and salts and are always clean), some glucose tablets and a packet of plain biscuits. Make sure someone knows you are ill. Check your blood glucose every two hours – you will probably have to increase your insulin. Keep sipping fluids and sucking glucose tablets. Nibble biscuits if you can. Call expert help sooner rather than later.

Foot care

Every year diabetic clinics wave goodbye to their patients as they set off on holiday, then anxiously await their return. Every year, despite huge efforts to prevent this, people return with ulcers or infections on their feet. A few lose their legs. The story is always much the same.

'I bought these new sandals in the market, real leather and ever so cheap, too. Then we went to look at the castle. It was very hot and a bit further than I thought and the road was all pebbly. The blisters didn't look too bad. I put a plaster on them. I thought the swelling was the heat. I couldn't rest them not with all that sightseeing to do, could I? They didn't hurt so I thought it was all right. They do look a bit red, now I come to take the plaster off.'

Take your chiropodist's advice before you go away. Never wear new shoes for the first time on holiday. Take your most comfortable shoes and avoid sandals – sand and grit combine with sweaty feet from the heat and all the walking and cause rubs and blisters and you can knock or cut your feet easily. Wear well-fitting training shoes with socks that are neither too big nor too small and will absorb the sweat. Make sure you take your foot care supplies with you. People with peripheral vascular disease (see page 141) and neuropathy (see page 139) are at special risk.

Have fun

By now you may be wondering if it is worth it. Obviously I have had to include a very wide range of potential problems but remember that most of them will not happen to you. Think ahead and be prepared. Then go off and enjoy your trip.

Useful phrases

These are some translations of 'I am a diabetic on insulin. If I am found ill, please give me two teaspoons of sugar in a small amount of water or three of the glucose tablets* which I am carrying. If I fail to recover in ten minutes, please call an ambulance.'

France Je suis un diabétique sur insuline. Si on me trouve malade, donnez-moi s'il vois plait, deux cuillières à thé de sucres dans un peu d'eau ou trois des comprimés de glucose que j'ai sur moi. Si au bout de dix minutes je ne reviens pas à moi, appelez une ambulance.

Germany Ich bin Diabetiker und brauche täglich Insulin. Finden Sie mich krank, geben Sie mir bitte zwei Esslöffel Zucker in Wasser aufgelöst. Der Zucker befindet sich in meiner Tasche oder Handtasche. Finden Sie mich ohmachtig, rufen Sie bitte einen Artz oder einen Krankenwagen.

Italy Sono un diabetico e sono attualmente sottoposto a trattamento con insulina. Se fossi colto da malore, per favore datemi due cucchiai di zucchero in una piccola quantità di acqua o tre delle pastiglie di glucosio che porto con me. Se non mi reprendo entro dieci minuti, per favore chiamate un'ambulanza.

Norway Jeg har sukkersyke og bruker daglig insulin. Hvis jeg blir funnet syk, vennligst gi meg to spiseskjeer sukker rørti vann. Det er sukker i min lomme eller min veske. Hvis jeg er bevisstløs eller ikke våkner, vennlist tilkall lege eller sykebill.

Portugal Sou um doente Diabético usando diairamente insulina. Se me encontrar doente deem-me faz favor duas colheres de sopa de açúcar em agua. Encontraro açúcar no men bolso ou saco. Se me encontrar inconsciente sem recuperar, faz favor de chamar um medico ou uma ambulancia.

Spain Soy diabético(a) y tomo insulina. Si usted me encuentra enfermo(a) temga la bondad de darme dos cucharillas de azúcar en

*Make sure you *are* carrying glucose tablets!

un poquito de agua o tres de los comprimidos de glucosa que llevo encima. Si no me recupero dentro de diez minutos, tenga la bondad de llamar un ambulancia.

Sweden Jag är diabetiker med dagliga insulininjektioner. Om Ni finner mig omtöcknad, var snäll och ge mig två teskedar med socker, gärna upplost i vatten. Det skall finnas socker i min ficka eller väska. Om jag är medvetslos eller ej svarar på tilltal kallapå en doktor eller ambulans.

Yugoslavia Ja sam dijabeticar i dnevno uzimam insulin. Ako me nadjete bolesnog, molim vas dajte mi dvije supene kasike secera rastopljenog u vodi. Secer se nalazi u mom dzepu ili torbi. Ako sam u nesvijesti i ne osvijestim ne, molim vas zovite doktora ili prvu pomoc.

SUMMARY

- Plan your holiday.
- Do not forget your diabetes travel pack.
- Do not forget your medical kit.
- Do not forget your out and about kit.
- Eat clean.
- Look after your feet.
- Enjoy yourself.

19

SETTING GOALS

Recently goals for diabetes care in Europe were agreed internationally. Because the St Vincent Declaration is such an important document it is quoted in full.

DIABETES CARE AND RESEARCH IN EUROPE: ST VINCENT DECLARATION

'Representatives of Government Health Departments and patients' organisations from all European countries met with diabetes experts under the aegis of the Regional Offices of the World Health Organisation (WHO) and the International Diabetes Federation (IDF) in St Vincent, Italy on October 10–12, 1989. They unanimously agreed upon the following recommendations and urged that they should be presented in all countries throughout Europe for implementation.

Diabetes mellitus is a major and growing European health problem, a problem at all ages and in all countries. It causes prolonged ill-health and early death. It threatens at least ten million European citizens.

It is within the power of national Governments and Health Departments to create conditions in which a major reduction in this heavy burden of disease and death can be achieved. Countries should give formal recognition to the diabetes problem and deploy resources for its solution. Plans for the prevention, identification and treatment of diabetes and particularly its complications – blindness, renal failure, gangrene and amputation, aggravated coronary heart disease and stroke – should be formulated at local, national and

European regional levels. Investment now will earn great dividends in reduction of human misery and in massive savings of human and material resources.

General goals and five-year targets listed below can be achieved by the organised activities of the medical services in active partnership with diabetic citizens, their families, friends and workmates and their organisations; in the management of their own diabetes and the education for it; in the planning, provision and quality audit of health care; in national, regional and international organisations for disseminating information about health maintenance; in promoting and applying research.

GENERAL GOALS FOR PEOPLE – CHILDREN AND ADULTS – WITH DIABETES

- Sustained improvement in health experience and a life approaching normal in quality and quantity.
- Prevention and cure of diabetes and of its complications by intensifying research effort.

FIVE-YEAR TARGETS

- Elaborate, initiate and evaluate comprehensive programmes for detection and control of diabetes and of its complications with self-care and community support as major components.
- Raise awareness in the population and among health care professionals of the present opportunities and the future needs for prevention of the complications of diabetes and of diabetes itself.
- Organise training and teaching in diabetes management and care for people of all ages with diabetes, for their families, friends and working associates and for the health care team.
- Ensure that care for children with diabetes is provided by individuals and teams specialised both in the management of diabetes and of children, and that families with a diabetic child get the necessary social, economic and emotional support.
- Reinforce existing centres of excellence in diabetes care, education and research. Create new centres where the need and potential exist.
- Promote independence, equity and self-sufficiency for all people with diabetes – children, adolescents, those in the working years of life and the elderly.

- Remove hindrances to the fullest possible integration of the diabetic citizen into society.
- Implement effective measure for the prevention of costly complications:
  - reduce new blindness due to diabetes by one third or more;
  - reduce numbers of people entering end-stage diabetic renal failure by at least one third;
  - cut morbidity and mortality from coronary heart disease in the diabetic by vigorous programmes of risk factor reduction;
  - achieve pregnancy outcome in the diabetic woman that approximates that of the non-diabetic woman.
- Establish monitoring and control systems using state of the art information technology for quality assurance of diabetes health care provision and for laboratory and technical procedures in diabetes diagnosis, treatment and self-management.
- Promote European and international collaboration in programmes of diabetes research and development through national, regional and WHO agencies and in active partnership with diabetes patients organisations.
- Take urgent action in the spirit of the WHO programme, 'Health for All: to establish joint machinery between WHO and IDF, European Region, to initiate, accelerate and facilitate the implementation of the recommendations'.

BUT WHAT ABOUT ME?

Dr R.D. Lawrence, himself diabetic, said

'In the successful treatment of diabetes the patient, the nurse, the practitioner and the specialist are often partners working together to establish the patient's health. In the long run the most important part, the melody, is played by the patient.'

He wrote that over 60 years ago. This book aims to give you some of the notes and harmonies you need to compose your own tune. But I hope it will also help you to use all the players and instruments in the diabetes orchestra.

The British Diabetic Association (BDA) founded by Robin Lawrence and H.G. Wells has formulated guidelines for people with diabetes. Again the implications of these guidelines are so important that I am quoting them fully.

ADULTS: WHAT DIABETIC CARE TO EXPECT

When you have just been diagnosed, you should have:

1. A full medical examination;
2. An explanation of what diabetes is and what treatment you are likely to need – diet alone, diet and tablets or diet and insulin;
3. A talk with a dietitian, who will want to know what you are used to eating and will give you basic advice on what to eat in future; a follow up meeting should be arranged for more detailed advice;
4. *If you are on insulin*: frequent sessions for basic instruction on injection technique, looking after insulin and syringes, blood glucose and ketone testing and what the results mean; supplies of relevant equipment; discussion about hypoglycaemia, when and why it may happen and how to deal with it;
5. *If you are on tablets*: discussion about the possibility of hypoglycaemia and how to deal with it;
6. A discussion of the implications of diabetes on your job, driving, insurance, prescription charges etc, and the need to inform the DVLC and your insurance company, if you are a driver;
7. Information about the BDA and its services and any local groups;
8. Ongoing education about your diabetes and the beneficial effects of exercise, and assessments of your control.

You should be able to take a close friend or relative with you to these sessions if you wish.

Once your diabetes is reasonably controlled, you should:

1. See a specialist nurse, doctor and dietitian at regular intervals – annually or more often if necessary. These meetings should give you time for discussion as well as assessing your control.
2. Be able to contact any member of the health care team for specialist advice when you need it.
3. Have more education sessions as you are ready for them.
4. Have a formal medical review once a year by a doctor experienced in diabetes.
   At this review:
   - Your weight should be recorded;
   - Your urine should be tested for ketones and protein;
   - Your blood should be tested to measure long-term control;
   - You should discuss control, including your home monitoring results;

208

- Your blood pressure should be checked;
- Your vision should be checked, and the back of your eye examined with an ophthalmoscope; a photo may be taken of the back of your eyes; if necessary you should be referred to an ophthalmologist;
- Your legs and feet should be examined if you are on insulin;
- You should have the opportunity to discuss how you are coping at home and at work.

The control of your diabetes is important, and so are the detection and treatment of any complications. Make sure you are getting the medical care and education you need to ensure you stay healthy.

WHAT PROFESSIONAL SUPERVISION SHOULD CHILDREN WITH DIABETES AND THEIR FAMILIES EXPECT?

1. **At and shortly after diagnosis** – initial assessment, treatment and advice:
- On the day of diagnosis the family should receive an explanation of the condition from a paediatrician of at least registrar status.
- Most children are admitted to hospital for a few days although where facilities exist they may be treated as an out-patient.
- When a child is admitted this should be to a paediatric ward where the nursing staff have an understanding about diabetes. Treatment should be accompanied by education on diabetes in general, injection technique and urine or blood testing.
- Senior medical staff should see the family daily to discuss diabetes and to deal with their anxieties and questions.
- A book such as the British Diabetic Association's *Handbook on Insulin Dependent Diabetes* should be available for the family on the ward.
- A dietitian should see the family on a number of occasions during their stay in the ward to ascertain previous food intakes, give dietary guidelines and provide written dietary advice.
- In those districts where specialist nurses in diabetes are available they will see the family during the stay in hospital and discuss with them the arrangements for further home visits following discharge.
- The family should be encouraged to join the British Diabetic Association. A member of the diabetic team should offer to phone the Youth Department of the British Diabetic Association so the 'Youth Pack' can be sent to the family.

- If a family support group exists the family should be told about it, so that they can be encouraged to make contact if they wish or have the choice to contact another family with a child with diabetes.
- The specialist nurse and/or dietitian should offer to make appropriate contact with the child's school.
- A member of the diabetes team will contact the Family Practitioner so that he is aware of what has been done during the child's stay in hospital. He will also be told of any possible liaison work with a specialist nurse who might see the family in their home. Although hospital management will continue in the outpatient department, most of the supplies can be obtained through the general practitioner and this also allows the child and his family to see the GP from time to time so that he is also involved in their management.
- The diabetes team should inform families of the circumstances in which the DSS Attendance Allowance is payable in respect of home supervision of children.

2. Initial control of the diabetes

- Instructions on the ward by the doctor, ward staff, specialist nurse and dietitian should include the following:
  – injection technique and advice on injection sites;
  – information and advice on injecting devices such as guns and pens;
  – the technique and interpretation of urine and blood testing should be shown to all children and parents;
  – the significance of ketones should be explained;
  – education will concentrate on the interaction of insulin, food, exercise, stress and excitement and how they affect blood sugar.

- There should be detailed discussion about hypoglycaemia with a simple explanation of its mechanism so that the family clearly understand its causes, symptoms and signs and treatment. Treatment should include the use of glucagon. The family should be told about the possibility of a hypoglycaemic convulsion and how this should be treated. This topic provokes enormous anxiety and time must be allowed for free discussion and reassurance.

- The 'honeymoon' phase should be discussed before the child

210

leaves the ward and the family given clear guidance about altering the daily insulin dosage as necessary.

- Ideally, direct telephone access to specialist advice through any member of the diabetic team should be available to solve problems as and when they occur. Patients should be told how they can get help quickly in time of need.

3. When the diabetes is reasonably controlled – long-term supervision

- The family should be seen by a specialist nurse, doctor or dietitian at regular intervals. Initially these should be frequent but eventually 3 to 4 times a year is usually sufficient. Whenever possible, children with diabetes should be cared for by a paediatrician with a special interest in diabetes and seen in a designated diabetic clinic.
- There should be sufficient time at visits to enable adequate assessment, general discussion, advice and education. At an appropriate time this should include discussion of possible long-term complications and their avoidance.
- Hospital visits should include the assessment of control by discussion of home blood glucose testing and the measurement of glycosylated haemoglobin or fructosamine.
- Height and weight should be monitored at each attendance.
- Discussion with young person and/or parents about general aspects of coping with life, counselling about alcohol, sex and contraception, driving, work prospects and possible long-term complications when appropriate.
- The transfer of the child's care to an adult physician may occur at any time after the age of 15. Whenever possible, joint clinics with the adult physician or some form of liaison will ease the change from paediatric to adult clinics.

4. Formal medical review

An annual examination should include:

- Blood pressure;
- Urine for proteinuria;
- Injection sites;

211

- Eye examination (this is generally begun some 5–10 years after diagnosis);
- Inspection of feet.

CONCLUSION

'The provision of comprehensive care for the child with diabetes and his/her family requires expertise and time and this is best achieved with a diabetic team.'

EUROPEAN PATIENTS' CHARTER

In 1991, the European Region of the International Diabetes Federation (IDF) and the St Vincent Declaration Steering Committee at the World Health Organisation Europe produced the first European Patients' Charter for people with diabetes. It has been circulated to all diabetes associations affiliated to IDF Europe. It is your charter – read it carefully.

YOUR GUIDE TO BETTER DIABETES CARE: RIGHTS AND ROLES

A person with diabetes can, in general, lead a normal, healthy and long life. Looking after yourself (self-care) by learning about your diabetes provides the best chance to do this. Your doctor and the other members of the health care team (made up of doctor(s), nurses, dietitian(s), chiropodist(s)) are there to advise you and to provide the information, support and technology so that you can look after yourself, and live your life in the way you choose.

It is important that you should know:

1. What should be available from your health care providers to help you reach these goals;
2. What *you* should do.

YOUR RIGHTS

The **health care team** (providers) should provide:

A **treatment plan** and **self-care targets**;
Regular checks of blood sugar (glucose) levels and of your physical condition;
Treatment for **special problems** and emergencies;
Continuing education for you and your family;

212

Information on available social and economic support.

Your role is:

To build this advice into your daily life;
To be in control of your diabetes on a day-to-day basis.

CONTINUING EDUCATION

The following are important items you should learn about:

1. Why to control blood glucose levels;
2. How to control your blood glucose levels through proper eating, physical activity, tablets and/or insulin;
3. How to monitor your control with blood or urine tests (self-monitoring), and how to act on the results;
4. The signs of low and high blood glucose levels and ketosis, how to treat them and how to prevent them;
5. What to do when you are ill;
6. The possible long-term complications – including possible damage to eyes, nerves, kidneys and feet, and hardening of the arteries; their prevention and their treatment;
7. How to deal with life-style variations such as exercise, travelling, and social activities including drinking alcohol;
8. How to handle possible problems with employment, insurance, driving licences, etc.

TREATMENT PLAN AND SELF-CARE TARGETS

The following should be given to you:

1. Personalized advice on proper eating – types of food, amounts and timing;
2. Advice on physical activity;
3. Your dose and timing of tablets or insulin – and how to take them; advice on how to change doses based on your self-monitoring;
4. Your target values for blood glucose, blood fats, blood pressure and weight.

REGULAR CHECKS

The following should be done **at each visit** to your health care professionals.
NB These may vary according to your particular needs.

213

1. Review of your self-monitoring results and current treatment;
2. Talk about your targets and change where necessary;
3. Talk about any problems and questions you may have;
4. Continued education.

The **health care team** should check:

1. Your blood glucose control by taking special blood tests, such as HbA$_{1c}$ or fructosamine (or fasting blood glucose in non-insulin-treated people); this can be done two to four times per year if your diabetes is well controlled:
2. Your weight;
3. Your blood pressure and blood fats, if necessary.

The following should be checked at least **once per year**:

1. Your eyes and vision;
2. Your kidney function (blood and urine tests);
3. Your feet;
4. Your risk factors for heart disease, such as blood pressure, blood fats, and smoking habits;
5. Your self-monitoring and injection techniques;
6. Your eating habits.

SPECIAL SITUATIONS

1. Advice and care should be available if you are planning to become or are pregnant.
2. The needs of children and adolescents should be cared for.
3. If you have problems with eyes, kidneys, feet, blood vessels or heart, then you should be able to see specialists quickly.
4. In the elderly, strict treatment is often unnecessary. You may want to discuss this with your health care team.
5. The first months after your diabetes has been discovered are often difficult. Remember you cannot learn everything during this period – learning will continue for the rest of your life.
6. You should receive clear information on what to do in emergencies.

YOUR ROLE

To take control of your diabetes on a day-to-day basis. This will be easier the more you know about your diabetes.

Learn about the practice of self-care. This includes monitoring glucose levels and how to change your treatment according to the results.

To examine your feet regularly.

Follow good life-style practices: these include choosing the right food, weight control, regular physical activity and not smoking.

Know when to contact your health care team urgently, including for emergencies.

Regular talk with your health care team about questions and concerns you may have.

Ask questions – and repeat them if you are still unclear. Prepare your questions beforehand.

Speak to your health care team, other people with diabetes and your local or national Diabetes Association and read pamphlets and books about diabetes provided by your health care team or diabetes association. Make sure your family and friends know about the needs of your diabetes.

If you feel that adequate facilities and care are not available to help you look after your diabetes then contact your local or national Diabetes Association.

NOW TAKE CONTROL OF YOUR DIABETES

This book and these guidelines will help you to look after your diabetes and to obtain the help that you need to do so. Gradually you will come to understand your diabetes. You will take command of it. But never be afraid to ask for help.

Remember: **you control your diabetes, your diabetes does not control you**.

Keep fit and enjoy life.

GLOSSARY

Acidosis Condition in which the blood is more acid than normal.

Adipose tissue Body fat.

Adrenal gland Gland found above the kidney which makes adrenaline and steroid hormones.

Adrenaline (American name Epinephrine) Flight, fright and fight hormone produced by the adrenal gland under stress.

Angina Chest pain caused by insufficient blood supply to heart muscle (a form of ischaemic heart disease). Also known as angina pectoris.

Angiogram X-ray examination of an artery.

Ankle oedema Swelling of the ankles.

Aorta The largest artery in the body running from the heart through the chest and abdomen. The aorta carries blood from the heart for distribution into other arteries around the body.

Arteriopathy Abnormality of artery.

Atherosclerosis Hardening and furring up of the arteries.

Artery Vessel which carries blood from the heart to other parts of the body.

Arthropathy Abnormality of joint.

Autonomic nervous system Nerves controlling body functions such as heart beat, blood pressure and bowel movement.

Autonomic neuropathy Abnormality of the nerves controlling body functions.

Background retinopathy The common form of diabetic retinopathy with microaneurysms, dot and blot haemorrhages and exudates.

Balanitis Inflammation of the penis.

Bed sores Ulcers in the skin and sometimes into deeper tissues over pressure points in someone lying or sitting in the same position for a long time.

216

Beta blocker Drugs which reduce high blood pressure, steady the heart and prevent angina. All the names end in -olol, e.g. atenolol.

Biguanide A type of blood glucose lowering pill.

Bladder Usually means urinary bladder. Bag in the pelvis where the urine collects before urination.

Blood pressure (BP) Pressure at which blood circulates in the arteries.

Candida albicans Another name for the thrush fungus.

Carbohydrate (CHO) Sugary or starchy food which is digested in the gut to produce simple sugars like glucose. Carbohydrate foods include candy or sweets, cakes, biscuits, soda pop, bread, rice, pasta, oats, beans, lentils.

Cardiac To do with the heart

Cardiac enzymes Chemicals released by damaged heart muscle.

Cardiac failure Reduced functioning of the heart causing shortness of breath or ankle swelling.

Carotid artery Artery which runs through the neck to supply the head and brain.

Carotid angiogram X-ray of dye passing up the carotid arteries into the brain arteries.

Cataract Lens opacity.

Cells The tiny building blocks from which the human body is made. Cell constituents are contained in a membrane.

Cerebral embolus Clot from another part of the body which lodges in an artery supplying the brain.

Cerebral haemorrhage Bleed into the brain.

Cerebral infarct Death of brain tissue due to insufficient blood supply.

Cerebral thrombosis Clot in an artery supplying the brain.

Cerebrovascular disease Disease of the arteries supplying the brain.

Charcot joints Damaged joints in areas of neuropathy (rare).

Cheiroarthropathy Stiffening of the hands.

Chiropodist Someone who prevents and treats foot disorders.

Chiropody Treatment and prevention of foot disorders.

Cholesterol A fat which circulates in the blood and is obtained from animal fats in food.

Computerised tomogram (CT scan) X-Ray which can take multiple very detailed films from different angles. Commonly used to look at the brain but whole body CT scanners are also available.

Congestive cardiac failure Impaired pumping of the right ventricle of the heart causing ankle swelling.

Conjunctivitis Inflammation of the conjunctiva (white of the eye and inner eyelid).

Constipation Infrequent and/or hard bowel motions.

Continuous ambulatory peritoneal dialysis (CAPD) An out-patient system of filtering wastes from the body of someone in kidney failure. Clean fluid is run into the abdominal cavity, takes up the waste substances and is run out again.

Continuous subcutaneous insulin infusion (CSII) A system for the constant pumping of insulin through a fine needle left under the skin all the time. Also known as an insulin pump.

Coronary artery Artery which supplies the heart muscle.

Coronary thrombosis Clot in an artery supplying heart muscle.

Creatinine Chemical produced by breakdown of protein in the body and passed through the kidneys into the urine. A measure of kidney function.

Cystitis Inflammation of the urinary bladder.

Diabetes mellitus Condition in which the blood glucose concentration is above normal causing passage of large amounts (*diabetes* = a siphon) of sweet urine (*mellitus* = sweet like honey).

Diabetic amyotrophy A form of diabetic nerve damage which causes weak muscles, usually in the legs.

Dialysis Artificial filtration of fluid and waste products which would normally be excreted in the urine by the kidneys.

Diarrhoea Frequent and/or loose bowel motions.

Diastolic blood pressure Blood pressure between heart beats.

Diet What you eat.

Dietitian Someone who promotes a healthy diet and recommends dietary treatments.

Diuretic Pill which increases urinary fluid loss. Diuretics are used to treat cardiac failure and most are also effective blood pressure lowering drugs.

Dot and blot haemorrhage Tiny bleeds into the retina in diabetic retinopathy.

Dupuytren's contracture Tightening of the ligaments in the palm of the hand or fingers.

Dysphasia Difficulty in talking.

Dysuria Pain or discomfort on passing urine.

Echocardiography Examination of the heart using ultrasound waves from a probe run over the skin of the chest.

Electrocardiogram (ECG or EKG) Recording of the electrical activity of the heart muscle as it contracts and relaxes.

Electrolytes Blood chemicals such as sodium and potassium.

Enzyme Body chemical which facilitates other chemical processes.

Epinephrine see adrenaline.

Essential hypertension High blood pressure for which no specific cause can be found.

Exudate Fatty deposit on the retina in retinopathy.

Fat Greasy or oily substance. Fatty foods include butter, margarine, cheese, cooking oil, fried foods.

Femoral artery The main artery supplying a leg. The femoral pulse can be felt in the groin.

Femoral arteriogram X-ray of dye injected into a femoral artery.

Fibre Roughage in food. Found in beans, lentils, peas, bran, whole-meal flour, potatoes etc.

Fluoroscein angiogram X-ray of fluoroscein dye passing through the blood vessels in the eye.

Gastrointestinal To do with the stomach and intestines.

Gastroenteritis Inflammation or infection of the stomach and intestines.

Glaucoma Raised pressure inside the eye.

Glomeruli Tangles of tiny blood vessels in the kidneys from which urine filters into urinary drainage system.

Glucose A simple sugar obtained from carbohydrates in food. Glucose circulates in the blood stream and is one of the body's main energy sources.

Glycaemia Glucose in the blood.

Glycogen The form in which glucose is stored in liver and muscles.

Glycosuria Glucose in the urine.

Glycosylated haemoglobin See haemoglobin Al$_c$

Guar gum A substance which slows the absorption of carbohydrate from the gut.

Gustatory sweating Sweating while eating.

Haemodialysis Artificial filtration of blood in someone with kidney failure.

Haemoglobin Al$_c$ Haemoglobin (the oxygen carrying chemical in the red blood cells) to which glucose has become attached. A long term measure of blood glucose concentration.

Haemorrhage Bleed.

Heart Muscular organ which pumps blood around the body.

Heart attack General non-specific term for myocardial infarction or coronary thrombosis.

Hormone A chemical made in one part of the body and acting in another part of the body.

Hyper- High, above normal.

Hyperglycaemia High blood glucose concentration (i.e. above normal).

Hypertension High blood pressure.

Hypo- Low, below normal.

Hypoglycaemia Low blood glucose concentration (i.e. below normal)

Hypotension Low blood pressure

Hypothermia Low body temperature.

Impotence Difficulty in obtaining or maintaining a penile erection.

Infarction Condition in which a body tissue dies from lack of blood supply – irreversible.

Insulin A hormone produced in cells of the Islets of Langerhans in the pancreas. Essential for the entry of glucose into the body's cells.

Insulin dependent diabetes (IDD) Diabetes due to complete insulin deficiency for which treatment with insulin is essential. Lack of insulin leads to rapid illness and ketones production. Juvenile onset diabetes. Insulin dependent diabetes.

Insulin receptor Site on the cell surface where insulin acts.

Intermittent claudication The intermittent limping caused by insufficient blood supply to the leg muscles.

Intravenous pyelogram X-ray of the kidneys showing the excretion of dye injected into a vein.

Ischaemia Condition in which a body tissue has insufficient blood supply – reversible.

Ischaemic heart disease An illness in which the blood supply to the heart muscle is insufficient.

Islet cells Cells which produce insulin.

Islets of Langerhans Clusters of cells in the pancreas. One form of islet cells produces insulin.

Juvenile onset diabetes Diabetes starting in youth. This term implies a need for insulin treatment. Type I diabetes.

Ketoacidosis A state of severe insulin deficiency causing fat breakdown, ketone formation and acidification of the blood.

Ketones Fat breakdown products which smell of acetone or pear drops and make the blood acid.

Kilocalories Cals or kcals. A measure of energy, for example in food or used up in exercise.

Kilojoules Another measure of energy. One kilocalorie = 4.2 kilojoules.

Left ventricle Chamber of the heart which pumps oxygenated blood into the aorta.

Left ventricular failure Reduced functioning of the left pumping chamber of the heart causing fluid to build up in the lungs and shortness of breath.

Lens The part of the eye responsible for focusing (like the lens of a camera).

Lipid General name for fats found in the body.

Liver Large organ in upper right abdomen which acts as an energy store, chemical factory and detoxifying unit and produces bile.

Macroangiopathy Macrovascular disease.

Macrovascular disease Disease of large blood vessels such as those supplying the legs.

Macula Area of best vision in the eye.

Macular oedema Swelling of the macula.

Malaise Feeling vaguely unwell or uncomfortable.

Maturity onset diabetes Diabetes starting when a person is over the age of 30. This term usually implies that the person is not completely insulin deficient, at least initially. Non-insulin dependent diabetes. Type II diabetes.

Metabolism The chemical processing of substances in the body.

Microalbuminuria The presence of tiny quantities of protein in the urine.

Microaneurysm Tiny blow-out in the wall of a capillary in the retina of the eye.

Microangiopathy Microvascular disease.

Microvascular disease Disease of small blood vessels such as those supplying the eyes or kidney.

Moniliasis Thrush.

Myocardial infarction Death of heart muscle caused by lack of blood supply.

Myocardium Heart muscle.

Necrobiosis lipoidica diabeticorum Diabetic skin lesion (rare).

Nephropathy Abnormality of the kidney.

Nerve Cable carrying signals to or from the brain and spinal cord.

Neuroelectrophysiology Study of the way nerves work.

Neuropathy Abnormality of the nerves.

Nocturia Passing urine at night.

Non-insulin dependent diabetes (NIDD) Diabetes due to inefficiency of insulin action or relative insulin deficiency which can usually be managed without insulin injections, at least initially. Ketone formation is less likely. Maturity onset diabetes. Non-insulin dependent diabetes.

Nutritionist Someone who studies diets. Nutritionists may be dietitians and vice versa.

Obese Overweight, fat.

221

Obesity Condition of being overweight or fat.

Oedema Swelling.

Ophthalmoscope Magnifying torch with which the doctor looks into your eyes.

Oral Taken by mouth.

-pathy Disease or abnormality, e.g. neuropathy, retinopathy.

Palpitations Awareness of irregular or abnormally fast heart beat.

Pancreas Abdominal gland producing digestive enzymes, insulin and other hormones.

Paraesthesiae Pins and needles or tingling.

Peripheral nervous system Nerves supplying the skeletal muscle and body sensation such as touch, pain, temperature.

Peripheral neuropathy Abnormality of peripheral nerves e.g. those supplying arms or legs.

Peripheral vascular disease Abnormality of blood vessels supplying arms or legs.

Photocoagulation Light treatment of retinopathy.

Podiatrist Someone who prevents and treats foot disorders.

Podiatry Treatment and prevention of foot disorders.

Polydipsia Drinking large volumes of fluid.

Polyunsaturated fats Fats containing vegetable oils such as sunflower seed oil.

Polyuria Passing large volumes of urine frequently.

Postural hypotension Fall in blood pressure on standing.

Potassium Essential blood chemical.

Pressure sores See Bedsores.

Protein Dietary constituent required for body growth and repair.

Proteinuria Protein in the urine.

Pyelonephritis Kidney infection.

Pruritis vulvae Itching of the vulva or perineum.

Receptor Place on the cell wall with which a chemical or hormone links.

Renal To do with the kidney.

Renal glycosuria The presence of glucose in the urine because of an abnormally low renal threshold for glucose.

Renal threshold Blood glucose concentration above which glucose overflows into the urine.

Retina Light sensitive tissue at the back of the eye.

Retinopathy Abnormality of the retina.

Right ventricle Chamber of the heart which pumps the blood from the body into the lungs to be oxygenated.

Right ventricular failure Reduced functioning of the right pumping chamber of the heart causing fluid to build up in the legs and ankle swelling.

Saturated fats Animal fats such as those in dairy products, meat fat.

Sign Something you can see, touch, smell or hear.

Sodium Essential blood chemical.

Steroid hormone A hormone produced by the adrenal gland.

Stroke Abnormality of brain function (e.g. weakness of arm or leg) due to disease of the arteries supplying the brain or damage to the brain.

Subcutaneous The fatty tissues under the skin.

Sulphonylurea A form of blood glucose lowering pill.

Symptom Something a person experiences.

Systolic blood pressure Pumping pressure.

Testosterone Male sex hormone.

Thrush Candidiasis or moniliasis. Fungal infection caused by candida albicans fungus. Produces white creamy patches and intense itching and soreness.

Thrombolysis Clot dissolving.

Thrombosis Clotting of blood.

Thrombus A blood clot.

Transient ischaemic attack (TIA) Short lived stroke with full recovery within 24 hours.

Triglyceride Form of fat which circulates in the bloodstream.

Type I diabetes see IDD

Type II diabetes see NIDD

Ulcer Open sore.

Ultrasound scan Scan of a part of the body using sound waves.

Uraemia High blood urea concentration.

Urea Blood chemical, waste substance excreted in urine.

Ureter Tube from the kidney to the urinary bladder.

Urethra Tube from the urinary bladder to the outside world.

Urinary incontinence Unintentional leakage of urine.

Urinary retention Retention of urine in the bladder because it cannot be passed.

Urinary tract infection (UTI) Infection in the urine drainage system.

Visual acuity Sharpness of vision.

Vitreous Clear jelly in the eye between the retina and the lens.

Vitreous haemorrhage Bleed into the vitreous.

USEFUL ADDRESSES

UNITED KINGDOM

Action on Smoking and Health (ASH)
5–11 Mortimer Street,
London W1N 7RH

Age Concern
Astral House, 1268 London Road,
Norbury, London SW16 4ER

British Diabetic Association
10 Queen Anne Street,
London W1M 0BD

British Sports Association for the Disabled
The Mary Glen Haig Suite,
34 St Osnaburgh Street,
London NW1 3ND

Cory Brothers (Erecaid)
4 Dollis Park,
London N3 1HG

Disabled Living Foundation
380 Harrow Road,
London W9

Health Education Authority
Hamilton House,
Mabledon Place,
London WC1 9BD

Help the Aged
St James Walk,
London EC1R OBE

In Touch
BBC Publications, PO Box 234,
London SW1

Keep Fit Association
16 Upper Woburn Place,
London WC1H 0QG

Medic-Alert Foundation
12 Bridge Wharf,
156 Caledonian Road,
London N1 9UU

Medical Shop
Freepost, Woodstock,
Oxon OX7 1BR

Optical Information Council
57A Old Woking Road,
West Byfleet,
Surrey KT14 6LF

Outward Bound Trust
Chestnut Field, Regent's Place,
Rugby CV21 2PJ

224

Partially Sighted Society
Queens Road, Doncaster,
South Yorkshire, DN1 2NX

Ramblers Association
1–5 Wandsworth Road,
London SW8 2XX

Royal National Institute for the Blind
224 Great Portland Street,
London W1N 6AA

The Sports Council (Greater London and South East Region)
PO Box 480, Jubilee Stand,
Crystal Palace National Sports Centre, Ledrington Road,
London SE19 2BQ

Synergist (Correcaid)
Genesis Medical,
115 Gloucester Road,
London SW7 4ST

AUSTRALIA

Diabetes Association of SA Inc
157 Burbridge Road,
Hilton, SA 5033

Diabetic Association of WA
48 Wickham Street,
East Perth, WA 6004

Diabetes Australia
33 Ainslie Avenue,
Canberra City, ACT 2600

Diabetes Australia
65 Davey Street,
Hobart, Tas 7000

Diabetes Australia (NSW)
149 Pitt Road,
Redfern, NSW

Diabetes Australia (Queensland)
124 Gerler Road,
Hendra, QLD 4011

Diabetes Education and Assessment Centre
74 Herbert Street,
St Leonards, NSW 2065

Diabetes Foundation (Vic)
100 Collins Street,
Melborne, Vic 3000

Diabetes Research Foundation of WA
Queen Elizabeth II Medical Centre, Hollywood,
Perth, WA 6000

CANADA

The Canadian Diabetes Association
(National Office), 78 Bond Street,
Toronto, Ontario M5B 2JB

UNITED STATES

American Diabetes Association
National Service Centre,
PO Box 25757, 1660 Duke Street,
Alexandria, VA 22314

Independent Living Aids Inc
1500 New Horizon Boulevard,
Amityville, NY 11701

Juvenile Diabetes Foundation International
432 Park Avenue, South,
New York NY 10016

National Association for the Visually Handicapped
22 West 21st,
New York, NY 10010

National Diabetes Information Clearing House
Box NDIC,
Bethesda, MD 20892

INDEX

Page numbers in *italic* refer to the illustrations

228

insulin jets, 89
insulin pumps, 89–90
insurance, 44–5, 155,
  196–7
intermittent claudication,
  141
International Diabetes
  Federation (IDF), 166,
  205, 212
intra-uterine contraceptive
  devices (IUDs), 173
intranasal insulin, 86
iron deposition, 37
islets of Langerhans, 30,
  86, 113
Isophane, 83

joints, 23, 138, 145
juvenile onset diabetes,
  33–4

ketoacidosis, 99, 180, 194
ketones, 99, 117, 180
kidneys, 10–11, 12, 132,
  134–6, 134
Kussmaul breathing, 21

labour, 176–7
lancets, 49, 51
languages, foreign, 203–4
Lawrence, Dr R.D., 207
legs, tissue damage,
  138–45
Lentard, 83
Lente, 83
libido, 137
ligaments, 23
lipids, 148
liver, 30, 132
lumps, insulin sites, 95
lungs, 21, 132

McLean, Teresa, 105
macular disease, 127
malaise, 6
marathon running, 187–8
medical checks, 153–4,
  211–12, 213–14
medical history, 17–19
medical kit, 199
menstruation, 118, 137,
  173

meters, 50, 51, 52
metformin, 65, 74, 76, 77,
  78, 187
minerals, 63
Minodiab, 74
mixing insulin, 94
Mixtard, 83
Monotard, 83
monounsaturated fats, 62
morning after
  contraception, 174
motion sickness, 195
mountaineering, 189
muscles: during exercise,
  179–80; facial, 124;
  fuels, 32; tissue
  damage, 140

nails, care of, 143
neck, tissue damage, 128
necrobiosis lipoidica
  diabeticorum, 123
needles, 87–8, 97, 200–1
nephropathy, 135–6, 135,
  148
nerves: examination, 22;
  muscle weakness, 124;
  tingling, 6; tissue
  damage, 139–40, 145,
  148, 150
neuropathy, 139–40, 145,
  148, 150
Novopen II, 88
numbness, 22, 139, 140
nurses, 166, 168

oestrogen, contraceptive
  pills, 174
operations, and
  hyperglycaemia, 119
ophthalmologists, 126, 167
Orabet, 74
oral contraceptives, 37,
  120, 174
oral hypoglycaemic agents
  see glucose-lowering
  pills
orienteering, 190
overweight, 34, 36, 42, 147

palpitations, 104, 106
pancreas, 31, 132;

inflammation of, 36;
insulin production, 30;
iron deposition, 37
pancreatitis, 133
parachute jumping, 189
penis, impotence, 137–8
Penmix, 88
pens, 88–9, 88, 91
periods, 118, 137, 173
peripheral neuropathy,
  139–40
peripheral vascular
  disease, 141–3
phlegm sputum, 21
phrases, foreign language,
  203–4
pig insulin, 83, 85, 112
pimples, 124
plasma glucose
  concentration, 13,
  14–15
polyunsaturated fats, 62
polyuria, 4
pork (porcine) insulin, 83,
  85, 112
postural hypotension, 21
pot-holing, 189–90
potassium, 63
pregnancy, 18, 36, 51, 80,
  118, 137, 172, 174–8
preservatives, insulin, 85
progestogen, contraceptive
  pills, 174
Protaphane, 83
proteins: in diet, 55, 60,
  61; in urine, 135
psychologists, 167–8
pulse rate, 21, 182
pumps, insulin, 89–90
Pur-in pen, 88
pyelonephritis, 134

Rapitard, 83
recovery position, 109, 110
reflexes, 22
renal glycosuria, 11
renal threshold, 11, 12, 54
restaurants, 157, 195
retinopathy, 126, 127–8,
  136, 148
rock climbing, 189
rowing, 188

230